The 10 Most Common Foot Problems We See

(How to Doctor Your Feet Without The Doctor)

by

Mark D. Sussman, DPM

and

Myles J. Schneider, DPM

Copyright © 2013

By Mark D. Sussman, DPM and Myles J. Schneider, DPM.

All Rights Reserved. No part of this book may be reproduced, scanned or distributed in any printed or electronic form without permission. Please do not participate or encourage piracy of copyrighted materials in violation of the author's rights. Purchase only authorized editions.

DEDICATION

For all the Podiatrists around the world who dedicate their lives

to keep us walking.

TABLE OF CONTENTS

CHAPTER	TITLE	PAGE
	Introduction	
ONE	Guidelines to Treatment	7
TWO	General Foot Hygiene	11
THREE	Ingrown and Thick Toenails	21
FOUR	Corns	31
FIVE	Callouses	42
SIX	Warts	52
SEVEN	Athlete's Foot & Other Foot Rash Problems	59
EIGHT	Bunions	66
NINE	Morton's Neuroma	74
TEN	Arch & Heel Pain	78
ELEVEN	Diabetes	105
TWELVE	Foot & Ankle Injury	117
	Acknowledgments	127
	About the Authors	128

Introduction

You do not need to know anything about medicine to be able to use this guide. The whole idea is to help you get relief from your foot and ankle problems. This is a "first place to look book" which will allow you to safely and often effectively deal with a problem. It could save you going to the doctor, but it will also alert you when it is indeed necessary to visit one.

Not all conditions can be self-treated. Read all instructions carefully. If you do not understand the instructions, are not certain what is wrong, or feel any reluctance to proceed with the recommendations, see a podiatrist or another qualified healthcare professional.

Disclaimer

The information, concepts, procedures and recommendations in this book are based on the authors' knowledge, expertise, research and opinions as well as their personal and professional experiences. The book is meant to be a guide to help you help yourself. The information, opinions, concepts, techniques and recommendations in this book are not intended as a substitute for consulting your physician or another qualified healthcare professional nor should you disregard your doctor's advice because of something you read in this book. Furthermore, the authors would definitely recommend you seeking professional care if you have any questions or concerns about any painful foot conditions you are experiencing in general.

FINALLY, IF YOU THINK YOU HAVE AN ACTUAL MEDICAL EMERGENCY CALL 911 OR AT LEAST CONTACT YOUR DOCTOR IMMEDIATELY!

The authors and publisher are neither liable nor responsible for any adverse reactions, effects, or consequences due to the use of any of the information, concepts, or recommendations contained in this book.

1. Guidelines to Treatment

1. *Do not attempt self-treatment if you have any of the following conditions:*

   - Diabetes
   - Circulatory problems
   - Infection
   - Queasy stomach
   - Allergies or sensitivity to any of the recommended materials and medications
   - Poor eyesight
   - Unsteady hand
   - If you injure your foot resulting in an open wound that is deep or very wide and/or bleeds a lot
   - If you sustain an injury and hear a pop, snap, or cracking noise followed by a substantial amount of pain, and/or swelling, and/or discoloration with or without bleeding
   - If at any time you have doubts or concerns about how you are progressing or your ability to deal with your problem yourself, seek professional care.

2. *Caution*

   - If there is swelling and/or black or blue discoloration that does not start to respond to the recommended treatment after 3-5 days, seek professional care.
   - If your problem is due to an injury and you have followed the recommendations for the first 24-48 hours, Rest, Ice,

Compression and Elevation (R.I.C.E.) and you still cannot bear weight on the foot, seek professional care.

- If there is swelling and/or black and blue discoloration that goes away after several days of reduced activities and appropriate self-treatment, but comes back again with just a slight increase in activities, seek professional help.

- If the pain and/or inflammation persist for more than 5 days after appropriate self-treatment, seek professional care.

- If the foot becomes very red, hot, swollen, and painful and you find it difficult to walk on it and/or if you see a red streak in your foot, seek professional care immediately!

- If at any time you start to feel sick, run a fever, have chills with or without redness and heat in the foot seek professional care.

- If you see a bump (hard or soft) that is under the skin and not a blister, seek professional care, immediately!

- If you have a "birth mark", mole, or growth on top of the skin, and it gets larger, changes color or becomes painful, seek professional care immediately!

- If at any time you have any doubts or concerns about how you are progressing or your ability to deal with your problem yourself, seek professional care.

3. **Precautions**

    - Know your limitations. If you attempt a self-treatment and it does not improve the condition, seek professional care.

    - Follow directions for self-treatment as written. Do not overuse suggested medications or procedures.

    - If during self-treatment you cause minor bleeding apply a styptic as directed to control it. If bleeding is excessive, apply ice and compression to the area and seek professional care.

- If you are instructed to use a heating pad for a specific problem, never use it when you are very tired and could fall asleep before turning it off. In addition, we feel it is best to use the low or medium setting to prevent irritating or burning your skin.

- Beware of frostbite. Do not use ice treatments for more than the recommended periods of time. Dependent on the type of modality you are using to ice your foot, you may want to wrap it in a towel to reduce the chance of frostbite.

4. **Preparation for Treatment**

  - Make sure any instruments you use are clean. Wash them in soap and hot water then rinse off with alcohol, Betadine Solution, or some other recognized antiseptic.

  - Make sure all materials and suggested medications are clean and up to date. To "sterilize" an instrument, carefully clean it with alcohol before using.

  - Scrub the entire foot thoroughly with warm soapy water and a terry wash cloth for at least one minute, and pat dry with a soft clean towel.

  - To prepare for soaking, dissolve any of the following in one gallon of warm water: two Domeboro tablets, two tablespoons of Epsom salts, or two tablespoons of a mild household detergent. Dip your feet/foot into the water and soak for ten minutes.

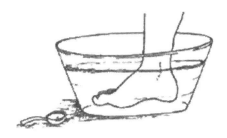

- Make sure to wash your hands thoroughly in warm, soapy water and dry them. If you wish you may wear a pair of plastic gloves as well.

- If someone else is assisting you or performing the treatment for you, then in addition to washing their hands, they should use plastic gloves.

2. General Foot Hygiene

- Inspect your feet daily. Check the tops, bottoms, in between your toes, and look over your toenails as well. Look for any discoloration in the skin, blisters, bruises, bumps, cracks in the skin, cuts, lumps, new corns or calluses, rashes, redness, heat, swelling or other signs of skin irritation.

- Wash your feet with warm water and soap. Be especially careful to clean between your toes. Try to use soaps that have glycerin in them as they are good for moisturizing the skin.

- Dry them carefully, especially in between the toes. Do not rub with a coarse towel.

- Apply a basic dusting powder or a medicated powder to your feet, especially in between toes, before putting on your socks.

- If you have problems with excessive foot perspiration and/ or foot odor, there are many sprays, powders, creams and/or "foot odor" insoles out there that can help alleviate this embarrassing problem.

- You may also have to change socks several times a day. Then, liberally powder your feet with a medicated foot powder or spray.

- You may have to change shoes daily. In addition, do not wear the same pair of shoes two days in a row if possible. Air the shoes out overnight and apply a disinfectant spray or powder into them before re-use.

- The SteriShoe Sanitizer is a product which uses ultra violet light to disinfect shoes in between uses. It has been shown to help reduce the amount of bacteria and fungus in shoes.

- If the skin appears to be especially dry (which often occurs on the heels and toes), apply a moisturizing product to them after the feet are dry. It is best NOT to use moisturizers with alcohol in them because the alcohol can cause evaporation of moisture from the skin. If you have very dry skin try using lotions with urea in them. Urea is an excellent moisturizing agent.

- Keep your toe nails trimmed by cutting them straight across. This should be done after soaking and cleaning your feet in some warm, soapy water or after a shower or bath. Then take a toenail scissor, nail clipper, or toenail cutter and make sure it has been washed in soap and water and rinsed in an antiseptic solution or rubbing alcohol.

- Cut your nails carefully straight across and file down any rough edges with a nail file or an emery board.

Cut your nails carefully straight across

- Dry thoroughly and apply a topical antibiotic to any nail that you may have nicked or that you can see a little blood (which can occasionally happen).

- Many people make the mistake of cutting the nail too short and this can lead to problems. The proper toenail length should be even with the end of the toes. If you cannot get into a comfortable position to cut your own toenails, then you should get someone to do it for you.

- Do not wear shoes without socks, especially for fitness and sport activities.

- Wear shoes whenever you are walking on city streets or any area where the surface is not clean and can be littered with broken glass, nails, and all types of other debris. These unclean surfaces can also lead to skin bacterial and fungus infections as well as warts.

- If for any reason you do go barefooted in a public place, make sure you wash your feet and inspect them carefully afterwards as soon as possible.

- Do not wear anyone else's shoes.

Socks

- On a daily basis, wear clean dry socks that fit properly.

- Socks and/or stockings should be between ½ - ¾ of an inch longer than the longest toe on your foot and not have any wrinkles in them.

- Your toes should have plenty of room to wiggle around.

- The best socks have breathable fibers like wool, cotton, or nylon blends.

- If your feet perspire a lot or they get wet during the day, change to a dry pair as soon as possible.

- There are some socks now that have copper and/or far-infrared blended into the fibers which helps wick away moisture and can decrease the chance of infection due to micro-organisms such as bacteria and fungus.

- Do not wear hosiery that has holes in them or that needs to be mended. The mending will often lead to the formation of seams that can be irritating to the skin.

- Do not wear socks with tight elastic top bands.

- Do not wear non-prescribed support hose because they may be too constrictive.

- Do not wear anything tight around the legs or ankles that might interfere with the circulation of your feet.

Shoes

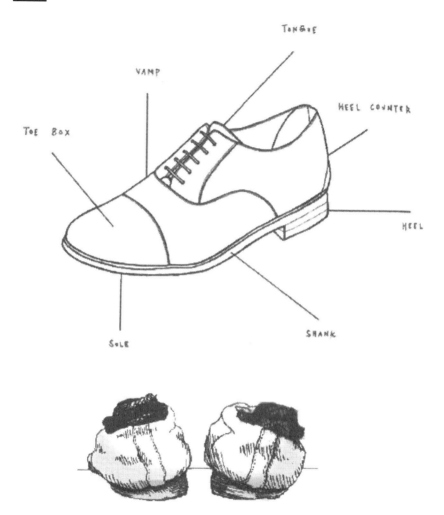

- **Worn down and/or old shoes can hurt you and should be replaced immediately.**

- Shoes must fit properly.

- Specific types of shoes should be utilized for different types of activities.

THE 10 MOST COMMON FOOT PROBLEMS WE SEE

- Go to a reputable shoe store where the sales people provide service to their customers and are knowledgeable about shoes, how to measure feet properly and how to match up the size they measured for you to the correct size of the shoes they have in stock. In addition, they should be able to help you be sure the shoes fit you well when you try them on.

  Have shoes fitted at the end of the day because your feet have a tendency to swell as the day goes on. If you have them fit in the morning or early in the day, they may be too tight by the end of the day.

- You should have both your right and left foot size measured in a standing position when purchasing new shoes.

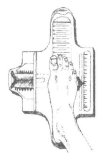

Stand on the foot being measured.

- Have shoes fitted while you are standing and try on both left and right shoes.

- Do not wear shoes made out of synthetic or leather substitutes which do not have pores and do not breathe well. Shoes should be made out of natural leather or out of fabric that allows for good ventilation. This will help reduce heat and perspiration in addition to allowing for a more comfortable fit.

- Be sure to wear your regular foot attire (double socks, foot pads, arch supports, extra shoe inserts, heel cups, and/or custom made orthotics) when doing this.

- You should not have to force a shoe on. No pinching or squeezing should be necessary.

- If this is the case, you need to go up another size and try them on again. The shoes should feel comfortable right away. You should not have to break in shoes from a comfort standpoint.

- When you try them on for the first time, make sure the back of your foot is against the inside of the heel counter of your shoe (arrows).

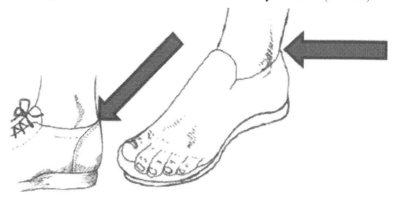

The heel should fit snugly

- You may have to gently tap the back of the shoe to get the heel of the foot in place. The heel counter should fit closely, but not too snugly either. Your heel should not be able to move or come out of the heel counter when stepping in place or walking forward. There should be only a slight almost unnoticeable, slippage or movement of the heel in the shoe.

- When standing up in them, check that you have a thumb's nail width between the end of the shoe and the end of your longest toe (usually about one-half inch).

THE 10 MOST COMMON FOOT PROBLEMS WE SEE

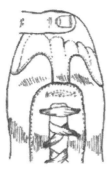 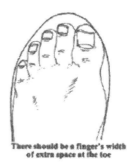

There should be a thumbs nail width of extra space at the toe

- Wiggle your toes while doing this to see which one is functioning as the longest and where it hits the shoe. It is not uncommon to have the second, or even the third toe be your longest. The toes should fit in the toe box area at the front of the shoes with enough room to allow free movement of all the toes without pressure on the ends, or in between them.

Make sure that it bends at the ball of the foot

- The ball of the foot should be located at the widest part of the shoe. There should be a pinch of material available (while standing) in the ball area of the shoe for a proper width fit.

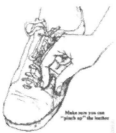

Make sure you can "pinch-up" the material

- The shoes should be about a quarter inch wider than your foot. It should not be so snug that you cannot do this. The foot should not be bulging at the seams here.

- Fully lace both shoes and try walking on them to see how they feel. If possible, try to find a non-carpeted area of the store to use when being fitted and trying out your new shoes. You cannot tell much about cushioning, support, or the true feel of the shoe when on a carpeted area. Just putting shoes on and not really walking or mimicking your fitness activity in them may be deceiving. The actual action and motions your feet will go through in the shoes can affect their comfort, and actually the way the shoe fits. A shoe itself will change in length when you go from just standing in it, as compared to flexing (bending) it.

- When it is bent, the shoe actually shortens itself, and if not fit properly, your toes will not have enough room at the end of the shoe. You may thus have to opt for a larger shoe size.

- Occasionally a pair of shoes will be defective. Therefore, be sure to examine the shoes closely, and if any of the following are not right, return the shoes to the store. Make sure:

- They are a pair. Always check the size and number of *each shoe before trying them on. Busy salespeople often throw shoes into a box that are the same style but not the same size. Buyers beware.*

- That they are symmetrical

- That the heel counters are equal in height and width

- That heel heights are equal

- That the inner arch supports are equal in size and in the proper place

- That there are no unusual seams or tears

- That the uppers do not slant inward or outward

- Human error... have you ever gotten dressed in a darkened room or closet and then gone to your workplace, school, etc. with two different shoes on only to notice it later in the day?

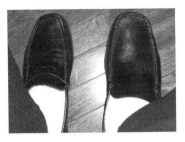

Two similar shoes: the left is a penny loafer and the right has a plain toe.

- **Refer to page 14, diagram of shoe for more information.**

- Different fitness/sports activities have different requirements of your feet and your body. If you are going to be involved in a fitness activity fairly seriously, it behooves you to get the appropriate fitness shoe for that activity. For example, you would not want to play tennis in a running or walking shoe, because tennis requires side-to-side motion and running or walking are straight forward motion activities. Therefore, tennis shoes focus on lateral support and stability. They are more durable and less flexible than a walking or running shoe. Trying to use a walking or running shoe for tennis will cause the shoe to breakdown quickly, will not support your feet properly, and can lead to injury. On the other hand, you would not want to use a tennis shoe for long distance running because the tennis shoes do not have the cushioning or the flexibility needed for running. You should go to a reputable fitness/running shoe store to get properly fitted shoes that are appropriate for your activity and your foot type.

- Different occupations have special shoe needs. If you are on your feet all day, and are required to do a lot of physical labor, you should purchase shoes with this in mind. Some work environments can lead to foot injury, and require special protective measures built into the shoes such as steel toes in work boots.

- In general, high heeled shoes are really not good for anyone's feet and certainly can cause problems when one already has foot problems or pain to begin with. However, if this cannot be avoided in your life then wear shoes with the lowest heel height as possible for you and try not to go above 2 to 2.5 inches in height. Also, try to find ones with the widest heels possible. This is especially important if you are an active, fitness enthusiast. It is also important to note that there are companies that offer quality, comfortable, stylish dress/work shoes that are designed to take stress off the feet.

Caution

Read through each chapter carefully and in its entirety before beginning any treatment. If you do not understand the instructions or if you are not certain what is wrong or if you feel any reluctance to proceed with the treatment recommendations, visit a podiatrist or other qualified healthcare professional.

It is important to remember that with any suggestion of surgery, especially elective (not life and death), a second opinion is always recommended.

3. Ingrown & Thick Toenails

Ingrown Toenail (Onychocryptosis)

What is it?

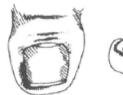

An ingrown toenail occurs when the side of a toenail cuts into the surrounding skin. The area becomes very sensitive to pressure. Continued pressure may cause redness, swelling and eventually infection. Nail pressure occurring over a long period of time may even lead to the formation of small, painful corns in the nail groove.

Things you may need for treatment

Adaptic (a non-adhering dressing material)

antiseptic

Band-Aid

Domeboro Tablets/Powder

Epsom salts

ice bag, cold pack or other modality for icing the foot

Merthiolate

mild detergent

nail clipper (straight backed preferred)

soap and water

styptic

topical antibiotic product

2X2 gauze pads

Preparation for treatment see page 9

Treatment

1. The only way to solve the problem of an ingrown toenail is to remove the ingrown part. Soaks and topical antibiotics are minimally effective without this step. If you do have an infection or inflammation around the toenail soaking and topical antibiotics may help reduce the severity of the condition. An ice pack held against the toe (for no more than five minutes) will provide some numbness.

2. To remove the offending part of the toenail...

    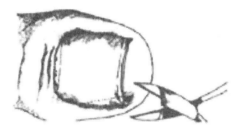

    Insert nail clipper under the nail border, as shown in the drawing. Clip out the ingrown toenail at a slight angle.

    Try not to cut flesh by keeping the bottom of the clipper as close to the bottom of the nail plate as possible. Hang in there! It is normal for this to be a little uncomfortable.

    Try not to leave nail spicules (pointed fragments) as they will tend to start the ingrown process over again.

3. Once the nail is cut, grasp the corner and gently pull it out.

THE 10 MOST COMMON FOOT PROBLEMS WE SEE

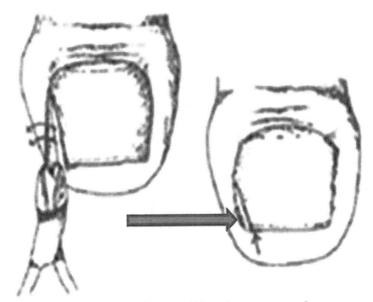

Arrow shows where nail has been removed.

4. Wipe off the area gently with soap and water on a gauze pad.

5. If there is bleeding, elevate the foot and apply an ice pack for ten minutes with light pressure. If bleeding is minor you may use a styptic. If it is excessive, apply ice and pressure and see a podiatrist or other healthcare professional.

6. During the next few days…until tenderness is gone, soak your toe for 20 minutes, twice a day in one of the following:

   Two Domeboro tablets dissolved in one gallon of warm water **_or_**

   Two tablespoons of Epsom salts in one gallon of warm water **_or_**

   Two tablespoons of mild detergent, such as Ivory Liquid or

   Tide, etc., in one gallon of warm water.

7. After soaking, apply Merthiolate (which will act as a drying agent), and/or a topical antibiotic of your choice, such as Neosporin. Then apply a piece of Adaptic (a non-adhering dressing material that prevents dressings from sticking to a wound) on it and cover with a Band-Aid.

When to Call the Doctor

If pain is not reduced after one day or if you have left a spicule (pointed fragment) or if you think you have an infection, see your podiatrist or healthcare professional immediately. If the do-it-yourself treatment provides only temporary comfort and the problem soon returns, you can have the ingrown part of the toenail permanently removed by a podiatrist through a minor procedure that is done under a local anesthetic with very little pain and almost no disability.

DON'TS

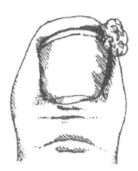

Don't stuff cotton or anything else under the nail edge. Cotton hardens and will cause irritation to the nail groove. This can give rise to corns in the nail groove often leading to pain and infection.

Don't waste time cutting V's, S's or any other design in the nail. It does not work.

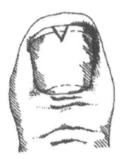

We don't recommend over-the-counter preparations.

They rarely work and may be dangerous.

Practical Pointers for Prevention

- Keep your toenails clean.
- Trim your toenails the way they are normally shaped, not necessarily straight across.
- Always leave the toenail a little longer than you think it should be cut.
- Watch for excessive shoe pressure.
- Do not wear improperly fitting shoes or socks (particularly those that are too short or too tight). This advice is of particular importance for children who are used to receiving "hand-me-down" clothing and shoes from older brothers and sisters.

Thick Toenail

(Onychogryphosis)

What is it?

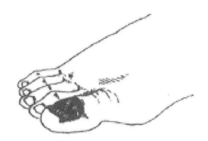

A toenail may become thickened and/or discolored because of an injury or fungus infection. It will be dirty yellow or brown in color, with occasional blackened areas. There is usually a white or yellow crust that flakes off the toenail, and under or around the nail a cheesy substance that may have a strong odor. The nail may be cracked and brittle. The most commonly affected nail is the large toenail.

Things you may need for treatment

antiseptic

Band-Aid

cotton

ice bag, cold pack or other modality for icing the foot

Merthiolate

nail brush

nail clipper (straight backed preferred)

nail file

salicylic acid plaster (40%)

soap and water

softening agent

topical antibiotic product

Preparation for treatment see page 9

Treatment

1. **The purpose of this treatment is *to reduce the thickness of the nail to reduce the pain*. This treatment will not cure the problem but may** allow you to live comfortably with it.

2. Cut the nail straight across with a nail clipper.

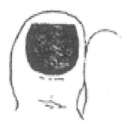

3. Take a clean file and a wisp of cotton and clean out the debris under and around the sides of the toenail. You may have to do this more than once.

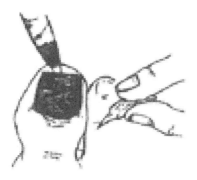

4. Cut a piece of 40% salicylic acid plaster, available at any place foot products are sold, to the size and shape of the nail plate. Put it on the nail plate with the plaster side against the nail and cover with a Band-Aid. Keep the toe completely dry for two days.

Caution: carefully read instructions on package before using.
Remember: try not to get the acid on your skin.

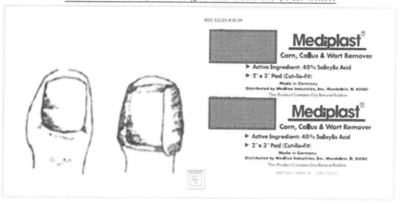

5. When you remove the plaster, take a nail brush or an old tooth brush and brush off as much flaky nail debris as possible.

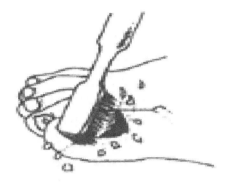

6. Then take your nail clipper and cut away as much of the nail as you can. File down any sharp points with a nail file or emery board.

7. Thoroughly clean the area with warm, soapy water and put on an antiseptic solution like Merthiolate.

8. Repeat the salicylic acid treatment for three to four times.

When to Call the Doctor

The salicylic acid treatment may cause a mild discomfort. However, if you have severe pain, swelling or infection, see your podiatrist or other healthcare professional immediately.

If the do-it-yourself treatment provides only temporary comfort and the problem soon returns, see a podiatrist or other healthcare professional.

DON'TS

Don't stuff cotton or anything else under the nail edge. Cotton hardens and will cause irritation to the nail groove. This can give rise to corns in the nail groove, as well as infection.

Practical Pointers for Prevention

- Keep your toenails clean.

- Watch out for excessive shoe pressure or tight socks or hose.

- When working or doing anything where you might accidently ***drop*** something on your toes, wear closed shoes to protect them. You should consider steel toed shoes if working with heavy objects.

- Change shoes and socks daily, as excessive perspiration, darkness and warmth are the prerequisites for getting fungus infections of the toenails. You can't find a better environment then the inside of your shoes for creating these conditions.

4. Corns

(Heloma Durum)

Corn on Top of Toe

What is it?

Most corns on top of the toe are due to hammered (contracted or claw-like) toes. The contracting usually occurs as a result of imbalances of bone structure or muscles that make the toe stick up higher than normal and cause pressure, both from the bone inside the toe and from the shoe outside.

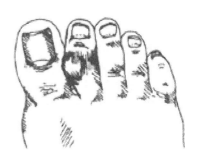

Things you may need for treatment

adhesive backed foam or felt 1/8"

adhesive tape ½"

Band-Aid

cooking oil

corn/callous file or "mildly abrasive tool"

corn pads, non-medicated 1/8"

lambswool

Meltonian shoe polish

moleskin

pencil

sand paper

shoe stretcher

soap and water

softening agent

toe spacers and/or toe separators

2X2 gauze pads

Vaseline

Preparation for treatment see page 9

Treatment

1. Dry the foot thoroughly and rub a few drops of cooking oil into the corn to further soften it. Take your finger and rub the oil into the corn.

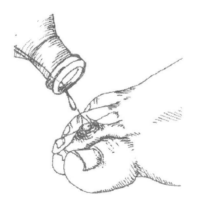

2. To provide temporary relief, remove the top layer of the corn.

3. Using a back and forth sawing motion, mechanically shave down the thick skin with a mildly abrasive emery board or other abrasive tool such as pumice stone, sandstone, sandpaper, or corn/callous file as shown. You can also make one from materials you can find around the house.

See page 41, for instructions.

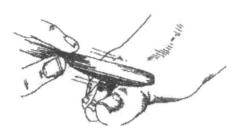

4. Make sure you stay on the overlying thick skin. If you can't see the line of demarcation between the corn and the toe, it might be helpful to circle the corn with a ball point or felt tip pen as shown.

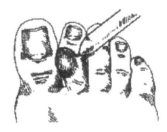

5. Corn and callous removal files can be purchased from the foot health products display at your local pharmacy, food store or online.

6. *DO NOT USE RAZOR BLADES, KNIVES OR ANY OTHER SHARP OBJECTS FOR THIS!*

7. Apply a commercially available *non-medicated*, adhesive backed corn pad, making sure it is thick enough to cover the raised portion of the corn and that the pad overlaps the corn by at a minimum 1/8 inch on all sides.

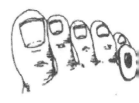

8. **Note: Hammertoes and corns that accompany them can occur on any toe and this padding procedure can be used on any hammertoe.**

9. To enlarge the hole, gently grasp the sides of the pad placing thumb and forefinger on either side of the hole and gently tug from side to side and the material will usually stretch. Do this carefully as the pad will easily tear.

To Make Your Own Pads:

1) Take a piece of adhesive backed moleskin, adhesive backed 1/8" felt, or adhesive backed 1/8" foam rubber. Cut a hole in it.

2) Trim to shape and stretch if necessary.

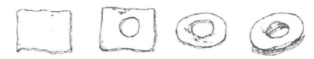

Apply as many thicknesses as you need to remove pressure (usually one is enough).

3) When the pad is in place put a daub of Vaseline ointment in the hole, then cover with a ½" square of gauze pad.

4) Wrap the toe gently with ½" adhesive tape or Band-Aid.

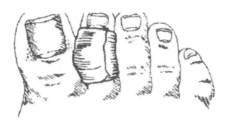

5) There are many commercially available corn pads for those of you that don't care to make your own. We recommend the non-medicated ones. Medicated corn pads can cause all kinds of issues. People with sensitive skin or medical problems such as diabetes should never use them. Check the foot health product display at your local pharmacy, food store or online.

When to Call the Doctor

If pain is not reduced after 3 days or you think you have an infection (if the area is red, warm or swollen) don't touch it yourself! See a podiatrist or healthcare professional immediately.

This treatment provides temporary relief but does not remove the cause. Permanent correction may be available from a podiatrist who can either keep the area trimmed down for you or straighten the hammertoe using a procedure that causes only minor disability and has been highly successful in achieving permanent "cure" for corns of this type.

It is important to remember that with any suggestion of surgery, especially elective (not life and death), a second opinion is always recommended.

DON'TS

- Don't use razor blades.
- Don't use any other sharp objects.
- Don't use medicated corn pads. They contain acids and can cause burns and infection in normal skin surrounding the corn.

Practical Pointers for Prevention

- Make sure you are wearing the proper shoe size with plenty of room in the toe box. You should be able to wiggle your toes. Remember that feet get longer as you get older.

- To relieve pressure, stretch the shoe at the spot where it covers the corn. You can also take the shoes to a professional shoe repair shop and have it done there or you can purchase commercially available shoe stretchers at these shops or online.

- You can put a broom handle into the toe box of the shoe and pull the shoe downward so that the end of the handle pushes out the fabric at the appropriate spot. Hold for ten minutes.

- To soften new leather shoes, polish with Meltonian shoe polish of proper color.

- You can use corn pads and/or shields that can be purchased from the foot health products display at your local pharmacy, food store or online.

Corn Between the Toes

(Heloma Molle)

What is it?

A soft corn forms between the toes when a bony prominence in one toe becomes "attracted" to a bony prominence on the adjacent part of the toe next to it.

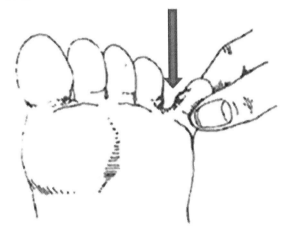

Over a period of time, with side-to-side pressure, they "hug" each other and a corn develops. The moisture between the toes keeps the corn "soft". Initially, these soft corns must be differentiated from an early fungus infection.

Things you will need for treatment are the same listed for corns at the beginning of this chapter (see pages 31-32)

Preparation for treatment see page 9

Treatment

1. Make sure the corn is well-softened with oil.

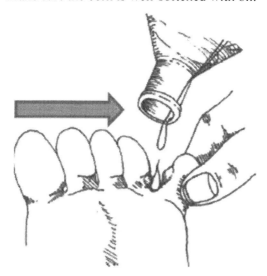

2. Remove the "top layer" of the soft corn to give temporary relief. Using your emery board or abrasive tool, file (away) the top layer of "dead" skin from the corn. Try to touch only the corn, keeping the abrasive tool away from the toe web (deep between the toes). If the corn is so large that it is located in the web itself do the best you can.

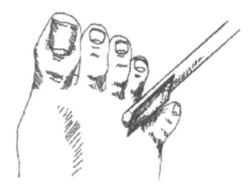

3. After you have removed as much "top skin" as you can, cleanse the area with a 2X2 gauze pad soaked in warm soapy water.

4. Rub Vaseline ointment into the areas you have just finished working on.

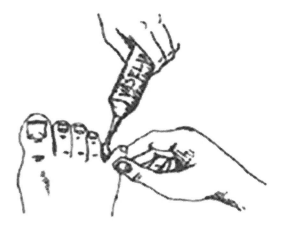

5. Insert a plug of lambswool about the size of a ball of cotton between the toes.

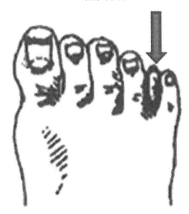

6. Use Vaseline ointment and lambswool daily to keep buildup under control.

7. There are many commercially available toe spacers/separators that work well for this. Check the foot products display at your local pharmacy or food store or order from an online source.

When to Call the Doctor

If pain is not reduced in one day or you think you have an infection (the area is red, warm and/or swollen), don't touch it yourself! See a podiatrist or another healthcare professional immediately.

In many cases, this treatment will provide temporary relief but will not remove the cause.

A podiatrist can keep the area trimmed down for you or may be able to provide a permanent correction by removing the bony prominence which caused the corn initially.

The removal is usually done with a local anesthetic and a minimum of discomfort.

It is important to remember that with any suggestion of surgery, especially elective (not life and death), a second opinion is always recommended.

DON'TS

- Don't use razor blades.
- Don't use any other sharp objects.
- Don't use medicated corn pads. They contain acids and can cause burns and infection in normal skin surrounding the corn.
- Don't put pads directly on top of a corn. This will only increase pressure and pain.
- Don't ever stick cotton between the toes. It will harden and cause increased irritation, just the opposite of what lambswool does.

Practical Pointers for Prevention…

THE 10 MOST COMMON FOOT PROBLEMS WE SEE

- Make sure you are wearing the proper shoe size with plenty of room in the toe-box to freely wiggle your toes.

  Remember that feet get longer as you get older. To relieve pressure, stretch the shoe at the spot where it covers the corn. You can also take the shoes to a professional shoe repair shop and have it done there or you can purchase commercially available shoe stretchers at these shops or online. Finally, you can put a broom handle into the toe box of the shoe and pull the shoe downward so that the end of the handle pushes out the fabric at the appropriate spot. Hold for ten minutes.

- To soften new leather shoes, polish with Meltonian shoe polish of proper color.
- There are many commercially available toe spacers/separators that work well for this. Check the foot products display at your local pharmacy or food store or order from an online source.

How to make your own *mildly* abrasive "tool"

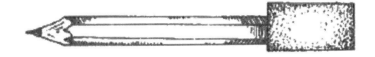

- Find a thin, clean piece of wood such as a tongue depressor, thin dowel, or pencil.
- Glue a 1" by ½" strip of medium grade sandpaper around its end.
- Allow to dry.

5. Callouses

On the Ball of the Foot

What is it?

A callous is a buildup of thickened skin that usually occurs on areas of extreme friction and pressure, such as under the bony areas of the ball of the foot.

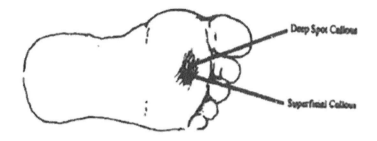

Usually a foot that is not aligned properly or not mechanically sound will "wear out" under continuous stress. What happens to the foot is like what happens when you drive a car with a poorly aligned front end causing the tires to wear excessively in certain areas.

The difference is that the foot protects itself by developing extra thickness in the skin in those spots where the skin might otherwise wear right through.

A "spot" callous is a deep, plug-like area of corny consistency located in the center of a more superficial, more spread-out callous. It is severely painful and can cause a limp in many cases. This particular corn-within-a-callous, as it is sometimes referred to, is caused by an abnormally depressed metatarsal head, or an overlong metatarsal bone. Since all the metatarsal heads are designed to bear an equal share of the weight load, if one is "too low" in the foot it will produce a pinpoint pressure point and a much greater stress in the skin on the bottom of the foot. You could achieve the same result from the outside-in if you taped a pebble onto the bottom of your foot and walked on it all day long!

Caution: It is important to be sure that what you are treating is indeed a callous, or a corn-within-a-callous.

Sometimes a wart, an ulcer or a foreign substance (splinter, glass, etc.) can resemble a deep callous in appearance and symptoms.

Things you may need for treatment

Adaptic (a non-adhering dressing material)

adhesive backed foam or felt 1/8"

adhesive tape 1 ½" to 2"

callous file

cooking oil

flat insoles (full length)

homemade balanced shoe insert

lipstick

magic marker or pen

moleskin

skin adherent spray

softening agent

Tincture of Benzoin

2X2 gauze pads

Vaseline

Preparation for treatment see page 9

Treatment

The same *general* treatment is recommended for all types of callouses. A few special suggestions will be given for each of the different types discussed.

1. Rub about 5 drops of cooking oil into the callous to soften it further.

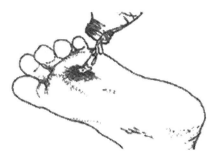

2. Filing down the callous

   - Using a back and forth sawing motion, remove the thick skin with a pumice stone, sandstone, mildly abrasive sandpaper (tool) or callous file.

   - Make sure you stay on the thickened skin.

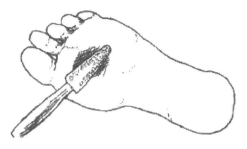

3. After filing down the callous, wipe off the area gently with soap and water on a gauze pad.

Take a piece of 1½" by 1½" adhesive backed moleskin, bend in half with sticky side up and cut a hole in it. If your callous is thick consider using 1/8" adhesive backed felt or foam for additional comfort. The hole should be wide enough to go around the callous leaving 1/8" border of good skin between the callous and the pad.

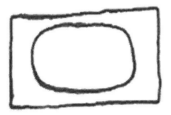

4. After the pad is properly placed on the foot, place a daub of Vaseline in the hole.

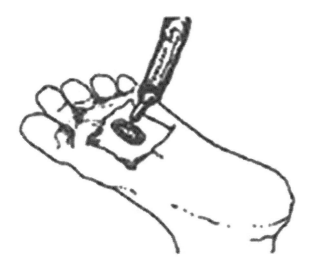

Cover with a 1/2" gauze pad (you will cut to size).

Cover this pad with 1 1/2-2" adhesive tape.

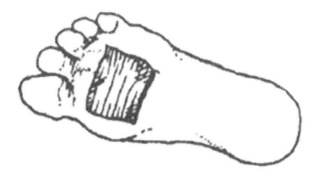

Note: If you are allergic to adhesive tape use non-allergic paper tape.

5. Once you have trimmed and medicated the callous, it is very important to pad pressure away from it. You will need the following additional materials. A skin adherent such as Tincture of Benzoin, and adhesive backed 1/8" foam or felt.

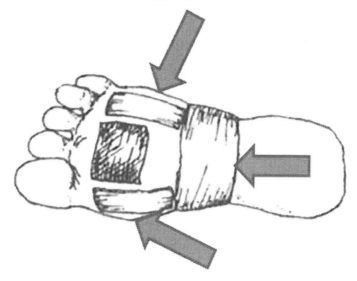

The arrows show 3 separate pieces of adhesive backed 1/8" foam or felt.

If the callous is in the *middle* of the ball of the foot:

- Prepare area with Tincture of Benzoin.

- Cut two strips of adhesive backed foam or felt ½" wide and 2" long.
- Cut 1 strip 2" wide by 2" long (see arrow pointing from the heel).

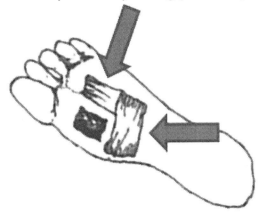

- For isolated callouses use combinations of the strips. The key is to redistribute the weight of the body away from the painful callous.

6. Keep pads completely dry for one full day after which it is ok to get them wet. We don't recommend total saturation with water, however. Don't swim or take baths and confine your bathing to a quick shower as long as pads are in place. You may use a hair dryer on medium heat setting to blow them dry after your shower. After wearing these pads for five days or less, carefully remove them as follows.

How to Remove Padding and Tape

- To loosen soak your foot in warm soapy water for at least 5 minutes.

- Always slowly remove the tape. When removing the pads or tape on the bottom of the foot, always remove in the direction of the heel; otherwise you may tear the skin.

- With one hand, firmly grasp the skin just in front of the pad or tape and with the other hand peel it slowly backward toward the heel.

- If you pull off the pads or tape in the wrong direction (side to side or from the back of the foot towards the front) and tear the skin there could be bleeding and pain. If this occurs, do not be alarmed but treat the wound as follows:

    - Do not cut the skin away, fold it down in place.

    - Apply ice, compression, and elevation for 10-15 minutes.

    - Once the bleeding has stopped, apply a topical antibiotic. Then place a piece of Adaptic (a non-adhering dressing material that prevents dressings from sticking to wounds) on top of it.

    Cover with a 2 x 2 gauze pad and tape down.

    - If you want to limit pressure to the area please use the padding described above.

THE 10 MOST COMMON FOOT PROBLEMS WE SEE

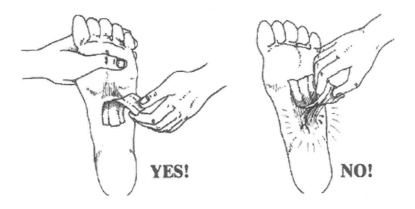

This bleeding should not be a major concern but if you are worried about it or if the skin becomes irritated from the tape and you are concerned, you should consider seeking professional care.

Remember, when removing the tape from the bottom of the foot pull it slowly toward the heel.

Liberally apply a medicated powder when dry.

For longer relief between home treatments, you can make a balanced inlay for your shoes to keep pressure off your calluses all day long.

Option 1: Go to a drug store or athletic shoe shop and pick up a pair of full length flat insoles.

Wear them for one week and your callouses will leave impressions on the insole, locating the areas of greatest stress and showing you the spots around which the insole needs to be built up to even out the pressure.

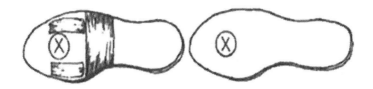

Or, instead of wearing the insole for a week, try holding it against your foot to feel where the callous hits. Mark an "X" at the spot with a marking pen.

Push in hard on the "X" until you feel your finger on the bottom and make a large circle around your finger. Use 1/8" adhesive backed foam or felt around the "callous" area (circle) just as you did on your foot.

With the insole in your shoe, the pads underneath the insole will redistribute your weight away from the callous and give you relief.

There are a number of commercially available insoles, but they may not provide enough pressure relief. These insoles we are recommending are fairly easy to make and you can enlist the help of someone who is "good with their hands" to help if you need to.

Option 2: Relieving painful pressure using the removable insert that comes with many shoes.

Color the painful areas of pressure on the bottom of the foot with lipstick.

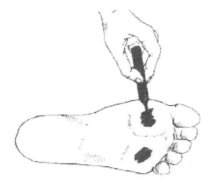

Put the full-length insole back into your shoes.

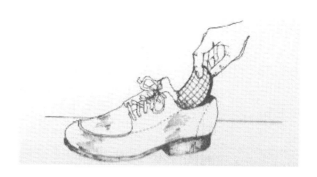

Walk around for 5 minutes (do both feet at the same time).

Remove the shoes and take the insoles out. Turn the insoles over. You should now be able to see and place 1/8 inch adhesive foam strips around the areas that need to be padded on the bottom of the insoles as shown.

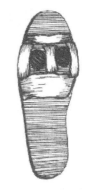

Wear this inlay in your shoe and you will walk in comfort. In fact in many cases your pressure points, over time, will disappear altogether.

If you need more support or if the insert wears down over time add more adhesive foam.

When to Call the Doctor

If pain is not reduced in two to five days, or if you think you have an infection (if the area is red, warm or swollen), don't touch it yourself! See a podiatrist or other healthcare professional immediately.

In many cases this treatment will give temporary relief but will not remove the cause. A podiatrist can keep the area trimmed down for you or may be able to provide a permanent correction by surgically lifting the abnormally depressed or overlong metatarsal bone. *In most cases the surgical procedure can be performed in an ambulatory surgery setting.*

It is important to remember that with any suggestion of surgery, especially elective (not life and death), a second opinion is always recommended.

6. Warts

(Verruca Plantaris)

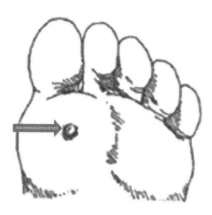

A wart is a virus infection that can occur anywhere on the body. It usually looks a little like a tiny cauliflower projecting from the skin, except when it occurs on the bottom of the foot. Then, due to the constant weight of the body, the wart starts to grow "into" the foot instead of "out" of it. Although warts are sometimes confused with corns and calluses, if you look at them closely you can see a well-defined border and little dark spots resembling blood vessels running all through them. They are also more sensitive to side-to-side pressure, while calluses are more sensitive to direct pressure.

They can be somewhat contagious and children are more susceptible than adults. They can occur as single warts or as a cluster forming one large wart called a Mosaic wart.

Things you may need for treatment

adhesive backed tape 1 & 1/2" to 2"

Band-Aids

Betadine Solution or some other antiseptic

Duct Tape

Freeze Therapy Kit (Cryotherapy)

skin adherent spray

salicylic acid plaster

soap and water

Tincture of Benzoin

toothbrush

Vitamins A, B complex, C, and E

Preparation for treatment see page 9

Treatment

1. There are several different options you have for self- treatment: salicylic acid, using good old-fashion Duct Tape and freezing them off.
2. Before going over these, you should be forewarned that warts tend to reoccur and can sometimes take a long time to get rid of. Over the years we have each treated thousands of people with warts and it is our opinion that the salicylic acid treatment is the most effective.
3. There should be no pain involved when treating the wart this way. It you do have some pain it is either due to the fact that you put the salicylic acid on the healthy surrounding skin or the wart is no longer present. When the wart is gone the skin will appear perfectly normal again. In either case, if this happens to you it is not really a serious problem. If the wart is still present and it is because the salicylic acid somehow got on to the healthy adjacent skin, then be careful and make sure it does not happen again. You

should stop applying the acid for two or three days and let the surrounding tissue get back to normal and then start again.

4. There is no limitation to the activities you can do with the moleskin and tape on. However, the acid will not be effective once it gets wet, so swimming would be out. If you do swim a lot, just do your best and keep the patches on as much as you can. It is also recommended that you re-apply the salicylic acid after a swim, bath or a shower.

5. Salicylic acid can be purchased wherever foot care products are sold. It usually comes on a square piece of self-adhesive backed moleskin impregnated with salicylic acid and will say 40% on the package.

6. There are many different brands. We are not recommending one over the other. The picture is for illustration purposes only so you know what you are looking for.

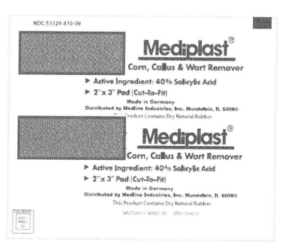

7. Cut a square of 40% salicylic acid plaster (about the size of the wart) and remove the backing exposing the self-stick surface.

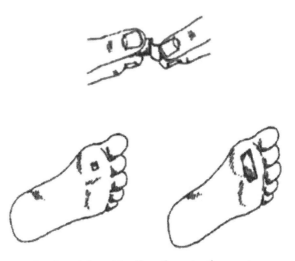

Apply sticky side directly onto the wart.
Push down and cover with Band-Aid or tape

8. Sometimes the pad and or the Band-Aid do not stick very well; if this is the case then you should use some skin adherent spray (like Tincture of Benzoin) to help keep it in place.

To do this, after putting the moleskin patch over the wart, spray adherent spray around it. Then apply either a piece of adhesive backed tape or a Band-Aid on top of it.

Remember, whenever it gets wet either by excessive sweating, shower, or bathing, it will no longer be effective. Therefore, keep the bandage on and dry.

9. *When you take the bandage off, do so carefully, after your shower or bath by removing the tape or Band-Aid pulling gently toward your heel. Do not remove the tape in a side-to-side or a down to up motion because you could irritate and/or tear your skin. See pages 48-49.*

10. Carefully remove the Band-Aid, tape, and plaster. The wart will have a whitish appearance.

11. Using a toothbrush which will become your wart brush, brush the wart vigorously for one minute and re-apply the moleskin patch and tape.

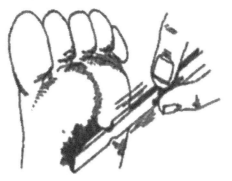

12. Do this for a week and check it to see if it is gone. If not, then repeat for another week.

13. Repeat this process every week until the wart is totally gone and the skin has returned to its normal appearance.

14. As mentioned above, this could take a while, meaning several weeks to several months.

15. If the warts are painful while you are treating them you can refer to the chapter on callouses pages 45-47 for suggestions on how to relieve pressure from them.

Other options you can consider:

- **Duct Tape** is another painless option people have tried with some success. You just cover the wart or warts with duct tape for up to seven days, and then soak your foot in water for a few minutes. Remove the tape gently toward the heel only (see pages 48-49) and use the tooth (wart) brush for one minute and get as much of the wart off as you can. Then repeat this process weekly until the wart(s) is/are gone.

- **Freezing** is called "Cryotherapy" where the wart is essentially frozen off. This method is available in drug stores, though they usually do not get as cold as the ones that a healthcare professional would use. If you decide to do this, follow the directions on the product you purchased. This type of treatment can cause some discomfort when walking for several days afterwards.
- If you are having trouble doing this on your own and find it difficult to self-treat your wart(s), then find someone to do it for you or see a podiatrist.
- Be sure to wash your hands thoroughly whenever you touch and/or treat your warts to avoid spreading them on yourself. To be safe use a pair of disposable plastic gloves when treating them. The person helping you should do this too because warts tend to be contagious especially among children.

DON'TS

- Use razor blades, knives, or any other sharp objects on the wart.
- Let the salicylic acid touch "normal "skin, if you can help it.
- Wear another person's shoes and socks in general but certainly if they have plantar warts.
- Use anyone's wash cloths and towels in general and especially if they have warts.

When to Call the Doctor

If there is no improvement after several months of consistent treatment or if the warts get more painful, or the wart or warts start to get larger and/or spread, seek professional care.

If you find it difficult to get into a good position to self-treat and/or you cannot find anyone else to help you treat it, then seek professional care.

If the foot becomes red, hot, swollen, and/or painful and/or you see a red streak on your foot, then seek professional care immediately.

If you start to run a fever, have chills, and/or do not feel well, seek professional care immediately!

Practical Pointers for Prevention

1. Do not go barefooted when in public areas like showers, locker rooms, and swimming pools. Try to wear flip flops or sandals as much as you can.

2. Change shoes every day. Do not wear the same shoes daily.

3. Children are prone to this condition more than adults. Check their feet periodically, especially during the fall and spring months. Early treatment prevents spread on yourself and to others,

4. Make sure you get adequate amounts of vitamins A, B complex, C, and E. If you have any questions about how much of these to take, consult with someone (a nutritionist and/or a healthcare professional) or some other reputable source for advice.

7. Athlete's Feet and Other Foot Rash Problems

What is it?

Athlete's foot is a very common superficial fungal infection of the skin of the feet.

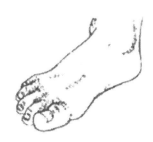

In the early stages fluid filled blisters can occur on the soles, arches, sides, and in-between the toes. The area can become very itchy, with peeling of the skin. Later these areas can become red, dry, scaly fissures. Dangerous secondary bacterial infections can occur if the primary (fungal) infection is not treated early.

Athlete's feet can be very resistant to treatment and can easily reoccur if not treated daily for a long enough period of time. Therefore, be patient, consistent, persistent, and pay careful attention to the **Practical Pointers for Prevention** section in this chapter.

Things you may need for treatment

Betadine Solution or some other antiseptic

Calamine lotion

cinnamon sticks

cotton socks

hydrocortisone cream

Ivy Dry

moisturizing cream

On Your Toes

plastic container or pan for soaking feet in

soap and water

SteriShoe Sanitizer (see page 11)

Tea Tree Oil

topical antifungal product (Desenex, Lotrimin, Tinactin, Reabsorb)

well-ventilated shoes

Preparation for treatment see page 9

Treatment

1. Apply topical antifungal creams or sprays like Desenex, Lamisil AT, Lotrimin AF or Ultra, Tinactin, Reabsorb (there are many choices) to the affected areas two times daily and once at bedtime or as directed on the label or product insert.

2. Cinnamon foot baths can help clear up this condition by slowing the growth of the fungi and other microorganisms that usually cause it.

3. To make the bath: Take about 10 broken cinnamon sticks and place in four cups of water and bring to a boil. Allow to simmer for about five minutes and then to sit for 45 minutes (do not put your feet into boiling water).

4. <u>Make sure the bath is lukewarm</u> and then bathe your feet in a plastic container or pan for fifteen to twenty minutes two or three times daily.

5. Another footbath that can be very helpful utilizes Tea Tree Oil. Add about twenty drops of the oil to a plastic container or pan with warm water in it. Soak for about fifteen to twenty minutes two or three times daily.

6. Once the acute stage is over (you have no more itching, no more symptoms, and it is not spreading any more) you can discontinue the baths.

7. If possible, do not use the same pair of shoes two days in a row.

8. After wearing a pair of shoes, air them out overnight and spray them with an antifungal spray or apply an antifungal powder (like Desenex, Lamisil, Lotrimin, Tinactin, or Reabsorb) to the inside of the shoes before re-use. You can also purchase a SteriShoe Sanitizer to help minimize re-infection.

9. Keep applying the topical antifungal cream for at least thirty days after the skin looks and feels like it is back to normal.

10. The microorganism(s) that cause this condition thrive in a dark, warm, moist environment (inside of shoe). If your feet sweat a lot, you need to try and control this. One good product to use to do this is called On Your Toes. It is a powder that you apply according to the directions for three days and then it will help control this problem for up to six months.

11. Wear well-ventilated leather shoes or sandals. Avoid wearing closed shoes that do not breathe well (have poor ventilation) like those that are made out of synthetic materials.

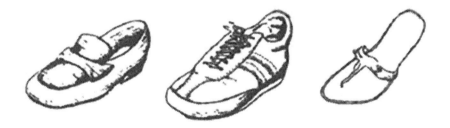

12. Wear white cotton socks as much as possible.

There are many other possible causes of rashes on the feet. The most common ones are:

Allergic Dermatitis (also known as contact dermatitis) can occur when you are sensitive to something that has come in contact with your feet like certain dyes or chemicals in shoes and socks as well as some clothing detergents. Poison Ivy is also in this category.

- If this is your problem, then apply over-the-counter hydrocortisone cream.

- Try to figure out what could have caused this and avoid it in the future.

- Practice good foot hygiene.

Diabetes-*Diabetics often have a tendency towards dry feet.*

- If you have diabetes, you should use a moisturizing cream on your feet at least once or twice daily to try and prevent dryness. If you do suffer with this problem, then apply the cream three times a day until it is under control and once it is, then twice daily.

- If your blood sugar is not yet under control, strive harder to get it so.

- Follow good foot hygiene for diabetics (See page 109).

Poison Ivy occurs when one comes in contact with the poison ivy plant and is allergic to it.

- Apply calamine lotion four times a day.

- Apply an over-the-counter hydrocortisone cream to decrease the inflammation several times a day or as directed on the tube.

- There are products that can sooth the rash and help dry it out faster like Ivy Dry.

- Wear socks and do not go barefoot especially when you may be in an area where there is known Poison Ivy.

Psoriasis-the skin on the feet and some other parts of the body with this condition can become very dry, scaly and flaky, and may bleed when irritated or scratched.

- Use a moisturizing cream on your feet twice daily.

- Bathe or shower in lukewarm water because hot water can be an irritant to the skin.

- Water can cause skin dryness. Therefore, you can add certain substances to a bath to help neutralize this, such as bathing salts and oils.

- Pat your feet dry before putting on the moisturizing product.

- Follow good foot hygiene.

When to Call the Doctor

- If you follow all the above recommendations and do not see improvement within two to three weeks or it seems to be spreading and getting worse, seek professional care.

- If the foot becomes red, hot, swollen, and/or painful and/or you see a red streak on your foot, seek professional care immediately!

- If you start to run a fever, have chills, and/or do not feel well, seek professional care immediately!

Practical Pointers for Prevention

- Wash your feet daily with mild soap and water, using a wash cloth or soft brush.

- After washing, dry thoroughly, especially between the toes.

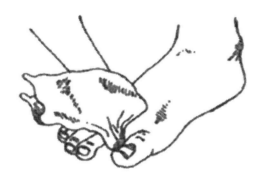

- If you are susceptible, use anti-fungal powder daily and apply liberally between the toes and in the socks.

- Wear socks that have some combination of synthetic fibers such as: Acrylics, Alpaca, Nylon, Polyester, and Wool.

- Avoid sweat socks as they are good absorbers of heat and moisture, and therefore contribute to the environment in which the fungi thrive.

- If your feet sweat a lot you can treat them with a product like On Your Toes, see number 10 under treatment above. You can also change your socks several times a day.

- Always wear socks or stockings when wearing shoes.

- Wear shoes that are well-ventilated like dress shoes made out of leather or well-ventilated fitness shoes as much as you can. Open toed shoes may also be a good option for women who have to look fashionable whether for work or play.

- Avoid shoes that are made out of synthetic materials like rubber or vinyl.

- If possible do not wear the same pair of shoes two days in a row.

- When removing your shoes after a day's wear, air them out for twenty four hours and spray them on the inside with an antiseptic spray such as Desenex or Tinactin before wearing again. You can also use the SteriShoe Sanitizer to prevent re-infection. Apply the SteriShoe Sanitizer treatment to a pair of shoes for forty five minutes after wearing them to accomplish this. Read the instructions carefully.

- Do not wear anyone else's shoes.

- Do not go barefooted, especially in public places like showers, gymnasiums, fitness facilities, and of course swimming pools.

- If anyone in the family has this condition, they should use their own towels and wash them daily. Shower stalls should be cleaned (disinfected) well after use.

- Everyone should wear sandals, flip flops, or something on their feet when in the common bathroom areas.

- Practice good foot hygiene (See page 11).

8. Bunions

An enlargement and/or misalignment of the first or fifth metatarsophalangeal joint

What is it?

The "big toe" bunion is an enlargement of the outside of the head of the first metatarsal bone. The big toe may be straight, but it is sometimes angled or pointed toward the small toe, subjecting the bony bump to a great deal of irritation. The skin and soft tissue around this bump 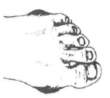 may become irritated and inflamed. The area may become red, hot, swollen and very painful. Continued pressure on this area can lead to the development of infection or the formation of corns over the bump.

The small toe bunion, or Tailor's Bunion*, is an enlargement of the outside head of the fifth metatarsal bone. The little toe is sometimes pointed in toward the big toe, causing irritation to the enlargement. The skin and soft tissue around this bump may become irritated and inflamed. This area may also become red, hot, swollen and very painful. Continued pressure on this area can also lead to the development of an ulcer, infection or formation of corns on the bump.

> *Before the advent of electricity, tailors who made clothes used a sewing machine that was run by pumping a treadle near the floor that was attached to the machine by a pulley system. Running these machines with their feet for hours at a time produced painful bumps on the sides of the operators' feet, thus the name "Tailor's" Bunion came into being.

Things you may need for treatment

adhesive backed felt or foam-1/8" and 1/4"

adhesive tape-1 1/2" and 2"

baby oil

bunion braces, shields, splints

cotton material 1" by 18"

elastic adhesive backed tape- 3" (Elastoplast)

flat insoles (full length)

heating pad

ice bag, cold pack or other modality for icing the foot

massage lotion

moleskin

over-the-counter anti-inflammatory medications

pillow

shoe stretcher

soap and water

soft polyurethane foam- ¼"

Tincture of Benzoin

toe straighteners

2X2 gauze pads

Vaseline

Preparation for treatment see page 9

Treatment

The goal of this treatment is to reduce the pain and inflammation around the bunion(s).

1. Make sure you are wearing the proper shoe size with both a wide and high toe box and wiggle room for your toes. This will help make sure that your shoes do not irritate your bunions. The shoes should feel snug but not tight. Loose shoes can also cause irritation from allowing your feet to move around too much. You may have to not only change your shoe <u>type</u> but also your shoe <u>size</u> to get the right mix. Remember that <u>feet get longer as you get older.</u>

2. You should use leather shoes because they are made from skins and just like your skin they breathe and are very forgiving.

3. To relieve pressure from the shoe on the bunion, stretch the shoe at the spot where it covers the bunion. You can also take the shoes to a professional shoe repair shop and have it done there or you can purchase commercially available shoe stretchers at these shops or online. Finally, you can put a broom handle into the toe box of the shoe and pull the shoe downward so that the end of the handle pushes out the fabric at the appropriate spot. Hold for ten minutes.

4. Consider using sandals, athletic shoes or open toed shoes until the inflammation and discomfort subsides.

5. Never wear the same pair of shoes for two days in a row. Shoes take 24 hours to both dry out and reshape (leather has memory) after a day's wear.

6. If you are still not getting relief after having tried these suggestions then do the following:

    - At the end of the day elevate your foot and place an ice pack over the painful area for 5 to 10 minutes.

    - Then take some baby oil or massage lotion or other similar friction reducing products and apply with a circular motion and gentle pressure for up to 10 minutes.

7. If this does not work then you need to further reduce the pressure by using some padding to disperse pressure away from the joint.

   - Apply Tincture of Benzoin to the irritated area.

   - Remove the irritation from the bunion by padding around it with 1/8" adhesive felt. Cut a hole in the felt a little larger than the bump and trim the circumference of the pad so that there is 1/8" to 1/4" width of padding all the way around the bump.

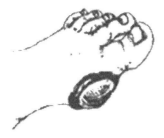

8. An alternative here is to use a commercially available "bunion shield".

   - Apply Vaseline into the hole, cover with gauze and tape down.

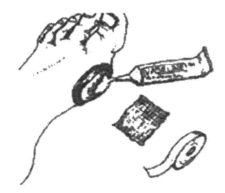

9. Make a "prehensile strap" as follows…

- Take a piece of 3"X 3" adhesive tape, Elastoplast (elastic adhesive backed tape) or moleskin and fold it in half, sticky side up. Cut into a "T" shape.

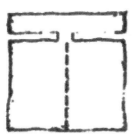

- Apply the top of the "T" around the base of the big toe and lock with tape.

- Pull the two bottom "T" flaps into place, covering the bunion. Pull the straight arrow piece into place first and cover it with the second curved arrow piece.

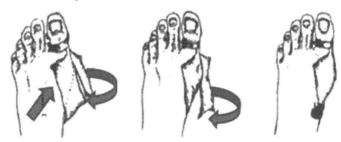

For further relief from pressure against the bunion joint, insert a piece of 1/4" inch thick foam or polyurethane foam or similar commercially available toe separating products between the first and second toes.

There are also many commercially available pads made out of different materials such as gel, rubber, felt that may be placed on or around the bunion to relieve pressure. These are available at the foot product display at your local pharmacy, food store or online.

Make an exerciser that you can use every morning to loosen up the bunion joint and make it more mobile.

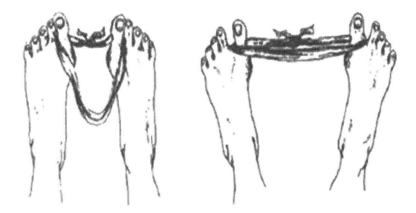

- Take a 1" by 18" piece of cotton material or thin rope.

- Tie a loop and place one end around each large toe.

- Keep heels on a flat surface, pull toes apart and hold for five seconds.

- Start by doing this pull ten times a day and increase one time each day until you get to twenty-five pulls a day.

- Once again, there are many products on the market that you can purchase to help do the same things. These categories include night bunion splints or braces, toe straighteners, specially designed socks and slippers.

- After you have tried the previous steps, if there is pain deep in the bunion joint or if there is redness or swelling around it, try the following:

- Get off of your feet except for necessary walking for a few days.

- Use local applications of ice up to 20 minutes two or three times a day.

- Follow the massage technique previously described.

- Take-over-the-counter anti-inflammatory medications as directed on the package for three to seven days. Follow closely the recommendations and possible side-effects on the package insert.

If you have a "Tailor's Bunion"...

- If your bunion is behind the little toe, place a pad around it, put Vaseline in the hole, cover with gauze and tape down as described in numbers 7 and 8 on page 69.
- The "exerciser" will not be of value for Tailor's bunions.

When to Call the Doctor

- If severe swelling, redness, heat and pain persist for two days with no relief, or if you see a break in the skin and/or are running a fever, see a podiatrist or other healthcare professional.

NOTE: *The treatments recommended in this chapter are aimed at providing relief for the pain and discomfort of a bunion. To actually get rid of a bunion, see a podiatrist or other qualified healthcare professional. In most cases the surgical procedure can be performed in an ambulatory surgery setting.*

It is important to remember that with any suggestion of surgery, especially elective (not life and death), a second opinion is always recommended.

DON'TS

- Don't wear a shoe with a narrow (pointy) toe box.

- Don't wear high-heeled shoes, especially when the bunion is in an acute (painful) stage.

- Don't wear socks or stockings that are too tight

Practical Pointers for Prevention

- Make sure you wear properly fitted shoes paying special attention to width and length.

- If you are an athlete, make sure you use athletic shoes designed for the particular sport you are participating in with a roomy toe box both in width and length. You should be able to wiggle your toes with your athletic socks and shoes in place.

- Once the pain is under control, you may wish to purchase a commercially available "bunion shield" to wear daily. Ask the pharmacist if you have any questions as to what to buy.

- To soften new leather shoes, polish with Meltonian shoe polish of the proper color.

9. Morton's Neuroma

Pain in the Front of the Foot

What is it?

Occasionally one or more of the small nerves in the front of the foot gets pinched between two metatarsal bones causing tingling, numbness, and/or pain extending from the adjacent toes into the front of the foot. This pain is especially noticeable if you squeeze the front part of your foot from side to side.

CAUTION: A painful burning sensation in the feet can be caused by many local (foot) as well as general body (systemic) conditions. Local pain can be caused by poor circulation in the foot, athlete's foot, a pinched nerve, or neuritis, such as Morton's Neuroma, described here. However, a general burning sensation can also be caused by diabetes, anemia, thyroid disease, alcoholism, and other conditions. Therefore, if you do not get relief with what is suggested, see a podiatrist or physician immediately.

Things you may need for treatment

adhesive felt-1/8"

flat "cushioned" insoles (full length)

flat insoles (full length)

heating pad

ice bag, cold pack or other modality for icing foot

Meltonian shoe polish

over-the-counter anti-inflammatory medications

shoe stretcher

Preparation for treatment see page 9

Treatment

1. When the burning sensation occurs, remove your shoe and massage the toes and front of the foot. Move the toes gently up and down. This usually makes the discomfort less and/or go away. When you do this and the pain is relieved this also is a diagnostic sign for neuroma. People who have neuroma(s) often describe this scenario.

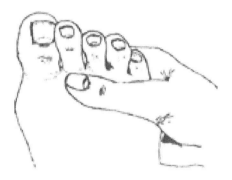

2. Do toe stretching exercises as illustrated. You want to bend all of your toes up and then bend all of your toes down. Do these 10 times twice daily.

Caution: if you get a muscle spasm in your arch when you move your toes downward, you can relieve it by immediately moving your toes up. If this happens take a few days off from this exercise and try again.

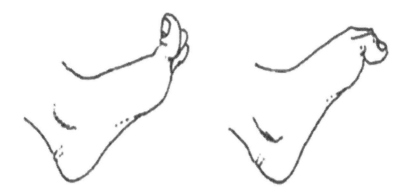

3. Wrap a heating pad around the foot two times daily for twenty minutes each time on the medium setting. If you have a home whirlpool bath, use it with <u>warm</u> water.

4. Place the triangular shaped pads cut out of 1/8th inch adhesive backed felt on the bottom of a flat insole to keep the bones that are *pressing against and irritating* the nerve separated. You can also put these pads directly on the bottom of your foot as shown here.

5. One pad is placed just behind the 1st and 2nd toes and the other is just between the 3rd and 4th toes.

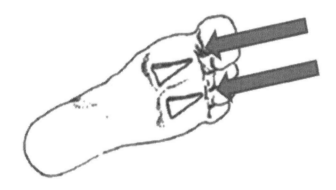

6. Take over-the-counter anti-inflammatory medications for three to seven days. Follow closely the recommendations and possible side-effects on the package insert.

Practical Pointers for Prevention

1. Make sure you wear properly fitted shoes paying special attention to width and length.

2. Wear shoes that have these features:

   - A large toe box, giving the foot plenty of room in the front (a narrow toe box will increase irritation).

   - Wiggle room for your toes is crucial.

   - Low heels, to keep pressure off the ball of the foot.

   - Laces, buckles or straps which will permit adjustment of width.

   - Wear thick, shock absorbing soled shoes. For thin soled shoes, you can add a flat cushioned insole, but make sure the insole doesn't cramp the toes.

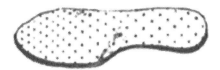

3. Make sure you are wearing the proper shoe size with plenty of room in the toe-box to freely wiggle your toes. We cannot say this enough! Remember that feet get longer as you get older.

4. To relieve pressure, stretch the shoe across the toe box. You can also take the shoes to a professional shoe repair shop and have it done there or you can purchase commercially available shoe stretchers at these shops or online.

   Finally, you can put a broom handle into the toe box of the shoe and pull the shoe downward so that the end of the handle pushes out the fabric at the appropriate spot. Hold for ten minutes.

5. To soften new leather shoes, polish with Meltonian shoe polish of proper color.

10. Arch & Heel Pain

Arch Pain (*Plantar Fasciitis*)

What is it?

The strongest ligament in the body is the plantar fascia. It is a fibrous band of tissue that starts on the bottom surface of the heel bone and extends forward on the bottom of the foot to just behind the toes.

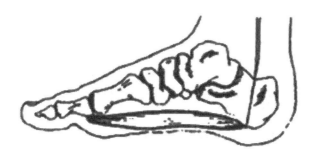

Its function is to protect the softer muscles and tissues on the bottom of the foot as well as to help maintain the integrity of the foot structure itself. With every step we take one heel or the other has to bear all of the body's weight on it. As we move, the stress load on the heel can be equal to up to twenty times your weight.

When the plantar fascia becomes painful it is called plantar fasciitis. For many years this term has been used to describe this painful condition which essentially means that the pain is due to inflammation of the plantar fascia. Recently, it is now thought that the pain occurs due to excessive tension or pulling on the plantar fascia where it originates on the bottom of the heel bone which leads to degenerative, repetitive micro-tears in the plantar fascia and ultimately the symptoms consistent with this condition.

This is now often referred to as plantar fasciosis. After resting and then getting out of bed in the A.M., the tissue contracts, while in bed and becomes very painful when first walking on it. The discomfort can usually be felt under the inside part of the bottom of the heel. It can range from very sharp to a dull, though intense pain.

One often feels stiffness in the feet and up the back of the lower legs when they first start walking and it takes a few minutes until it starts to loosen up a bit. The pain can extend into the inside bottom of the arch. It is relieved by getting off of one's feet but if you rest awhile it can be very painful once you stand and start moving again. The pain can be exacerbated by walking on hard surfaces, walking fast, carrying heavy objects, and participating in a variety of fitness activities. If left untreated or allowed to go on too long, it can become very disabling.

The plantar fascia can occasionally become torn or ruptured. This usually occurs during some type of fitness/ athletic activity and people often say they could hear and feel a popping type of noise. A ruptured plantar fascia is most often accompanied by significant pain, swelling, and discoloration. It is also very difficult to bear weight on it.

If you think this might be what has just happened to you, you need to seek professional care.

If you have to wait for several hours or to the next day or so, follow the recommendations for Rest, Ice, Compression and Elevation (see pages 119-123) until you can have it professionally evaluated. See items one and two in treatment recommendations below.

Things you may need for treatment

adhesive backed felt 1/4"

adhesive tape 1" and 1-1/2" to 2"

arch support

baby oil

Betadine Solution or some other antiseptic

flat store bought insole

foot massage product, foot roller, ball, or can of food

foot support insole

gauze pads (2x2)

heel cups (gel or rubber made)

ice bag, cold pack, or other modality used for icing the foot.

massage lotion

over-the-counter anti-inflammatories

pillows

plantar fascial brace

plantar fascial strap

powder or paraffin wax

removable arch pad or brace

removable elastic arch binder, pad, and/or brace

skin adherent spray

soap and water

supportive shoes

towel or Theraband

Vaseline

Preparation for treatment see page 9

Treatment

1. **Rest and Elevation:** You should rest and elevate your feet as much as possible for the first 24-48 hours. After 48 hours, if you still feel pain, do not walk any more than necessary or participate in weight bearing, fitness activities. Then continue to rest and elevate your feet whenever you can.

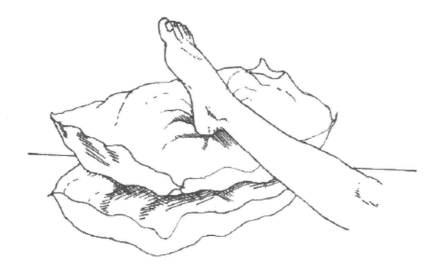

2. **Apply ice** 10-20 minutes at a time at least three times a day when possible for the first 48 hours, to reduce pain, swelling, and inflammation. This can be done using a cup of ice, a towel wrapped around a plastic bag of crushed ice, an ice bag, cold pack or a bag of frozen vegetables. You should also elevate the foot on two pillows and if you have a good deal of swelling use compression as well.

ICING Suggestions

Some examples are shown here:

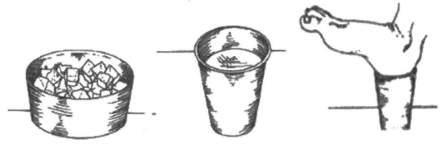

3. **Ice and Compression:** (Ace-Type Bandage)

- Arrow shows ice under compression bandage.

- *Do not place ice directly on skin.* Put a thin cloth barrier such as two large gauze pads then put cubes or crushed ice in a sandwich sized plastic baggie. Hold on area with Ace wrap (large arrow).

- *The picture below is an example. If you have arch or heel pain the ice will be placed in those areas...smaller arrows*

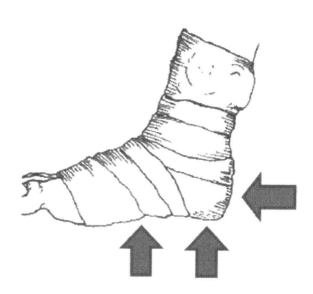

4. Do not go barefooted until the pain has been totally gone for a week or so.

5. Wear some good, shock absorbing, supportive shoes as much as possible both around the house, when you go out and even at work if allowed. The best type of shoe for this would be a quality fitness shoe.

6. Avoid slippers, thongs, sandals, canvas, and deck shoes.

7. Mechanical stress to the bottom of the heel and arch needs to be removed or at least decreased. There are several ways to do this. One of the best ways is to apply what is called a "low dye taping technique to the foot. Here's how…

- Use a skin adherent spray over the area of the foot to be taped.

- Cut three or four pieces of 1-1/2" or 2" adhesive tape, each five to six inches long. Anchor each piece along the outside border of the foot and pull inward and upward with plenty of tension to support the arch. Start with the first piece of tape about one inch in front of the heel.

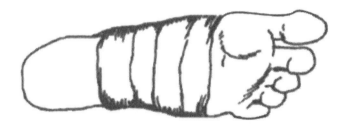

- If this does not take some of the pain away or provide enough support, carefully remove the tape(see page 48-49) if it is still on then start with two retention straps as follows:

- Clean the foot in preparation for taping again and use the tape adherent spray over the area to be taped again as well.

- Cut three strips of 1" adhesive tape, approximately 8-12" long, depending upon the size of your foot.

- To avoid irritation to the back of the heel, before taping, place some Vaseline in that area and cover it with a piece or two of 2X2 gauze.*See arrow below...

- Place one end of the tape along the outside border of the foot, about one inch behind the little toe. Following the outside border of the foot, take the tape behind the heel and around the other side of the foot, ending about one inch behind the big toe. Before placing the tape down and in place on the foot, point your toes downward to raise your arch up then smooth the tape down.

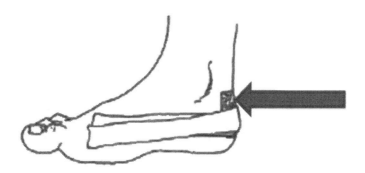

- Arrow pointing to gauze pad and Vaseline on back of heel for irritation prevention.

- After two retention straps are on, place the arch straps as described above.

- Then apply the third retention strap the same way as the first two.

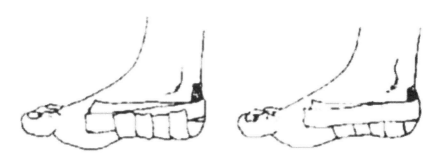

- All of this is finally anchored securely by placing one or two strips of 1-1/2 or 2" wide adhesive tape on the top of the foot and ending underneath the arch on each side. To prevent irritation to the skin or blistering, apply a generous amount of Vaseline here and then cover with two pieces of 2x2 gauze, before applying these retention straps.

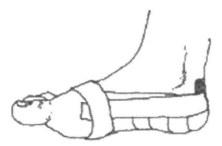

- After taping is in place, dust the taping liberally with powder to prevent sticking to socks and twisting of tape. As an alternative, rub a piece of paraffin wax over the tape.

- **It is important to note when using one of these taping techniques that there is no space allowed (no skin showing in between strips of tape). Overlap one piece of tape over the other as you put them on otherwise you can irritate the skin, get blisters, and/or cause small cuts in the skin.**

- If the taping alone does not seem to help enough, then try using a 1/8" or ¼" adhesive backed felt arch pad cut to the contour of your arch. Prepare the skin for taping as described above. Secure the arch pad on the foot first and then cover with either one of the aforementioned taping techniques.

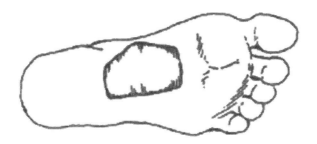

- To get even more support for both the heel and arch you can take a piece of 1/8" or ¼" adhesive backed felt and cut it in the shape of a "J" to cushion both the arch and heel. Prepare the skin for taping, secure the "J" shaped pad to the foot, and then cover with one of the aforementioned taping techniques.

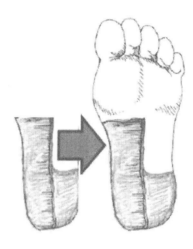

Placement of "J" pad on the bottom of the left foot

8. **The following are some examples of different things you may have experienced during the time you were caring for your specific problem(s), followed by some of the options available to you.**

- If you taped your foot (with or without padding) and you felt complete relief of your symptoms but they returned when you took the tape and pads off-

- If you taped your foot (with or without padding) and you noted some improvement of your symptoms but the foot felt as bad as it did once the taping and padding was removed-

- If you had some or complete relief with the symptoms with the taping (with or without the padding) and noticed the symptoms again without it but do not want to have to keep taping and padding your foot-

- If you do not want to try taping or padding at all-

- If you did not notice any difference with the tapping and padding-

- If you found the taping (with or without padding) significantly to somewhat helpful but the skin on your foot is getting irritated from the repetitive taping-

- If after the severe stage is under control (this may take up to a month or two of the taping and padding) you will want to keep the condition controlled by using something to support the heel and arch of your feet-

9. **Here are some additional options that are available to you:**

    - An arch elastic wrap or binder

    - A removable arch pad or brace

    - A plantar fascial strap

    - An arch support

    - Many people find gel or rubber made heel cups helpful as well. We recommend if you are going to use them, wear them over your arch supports or foot support insoles.

10. You can make your own foot support insole yourself.

To make your own Foot Support Insole:

- Purchase a pair of full length flat insoles.

- On the bottom of the insole, mark the center of the heel (bisect with a pen).

- Mark the widest portion (across the ball joint), bisecting the ball width-wise (extend from behind the big toe to just behind the little toe). Mark another line parallel and one inch behind the ball joint line as shown (both of these lines will course slightly diagonally across the bottom of the inlay).

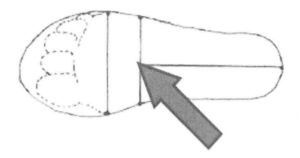

- Bisect the second line, extending the heel bisection line until the two lines intersect

  (see arrow above).

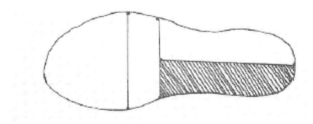

- Fill the entire *inside* portion of the inlay between the lines with 1/8 inch to 1/4 inch adhesive backed foam or felt (this is also referred to as a "varus" wedge).

- Bevel the edges of the foam or felt with a scissors or a file.

- You can also use a "J" pad in the same way (see page 86).

- Putting these inserts in your shoes will reduce the pull on the plantar fascia and can provide considerable relief.

- ***WHENEVER YOU USE AN ARCH SUPPORT OR FOOT SUPPORT INSOLE, AND/OR HEEL CUPS, YOU NEED TO HAVE <u>ONE FOR BOTH FEET</u> SO AS NOT TO CAUSE ASSYMETRY OR CREATE A LIMB LENGTH DISCREPANCY.***

11. **Medication:** Take over-the-counter anti-inflammatory medications for three to seven days. Follow closely the recommendations and possible side-effects on the package insert.

12. **Massaging** the bottom of the heel and arch can also help to alleviate the symptoms. Massaging the bottom of the foot and arch can be done manually.

- Massaging the bottom of the foot can also be done by pushing down, then rolling the arch of the foot forward and backwards over a tennis ball, a can of food or juice, a rolling pin, or you can purchase a number of foot massage products.

- Massage the bottom of the foot for 2-5 minutes up to three times daily until the pain has improved or gone away.

- A bottle of cold water used for an arch massage is effective.

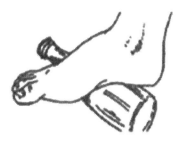
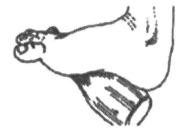

- Tightness in the calf muscles can often contribute to plantar fasciitis. Therefore, massaging the calf muscles in the back of the leg for 2-5 minutes up to three times a day can also help.

- There is a deep tissue massage technique that you can incorporate when you are massaging the bottom of your foot and calf muscles to try and alleviate the painful knots or trigger points (hyperirritable painful knots in muscles) that can contribute to, if not be the primary cause of this painful condition.

- Below is the location of these trigger points. See the **"X's"**. Using your thumb, press down *very hard* on these areas and hold for six seconds, then gradually release the stress and repeat five to ten times at least once a day. You may need to press down several times moving your thumb around the X marked areas until you locate the *most* painful spots. These are the areas to press on. We know it sounds silly to press on painful spots to relieve pain, but it works.

- If you are queasy doing this, you may have someone else do it.

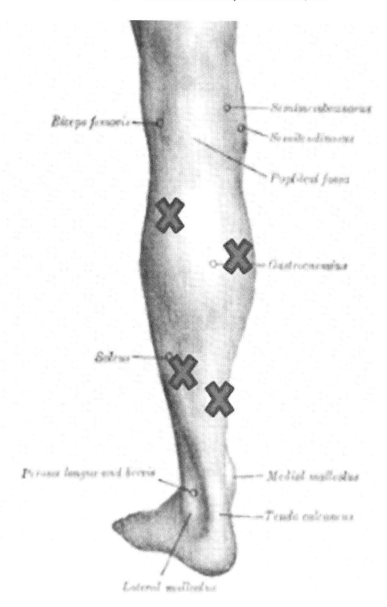

X marks the trigger points.

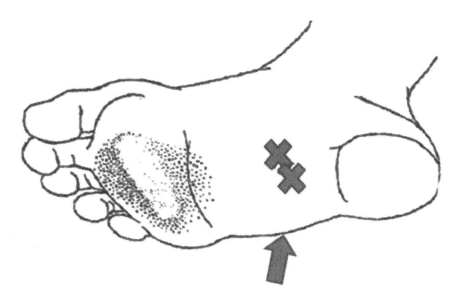

X marks the trigger points.

13. **Stretching** the back of the lower and upper legs, as well as the low back can also help eliminate this painful condition. As a matter of fact, it is highly recommended that you continue doing this once a day, after the symptoms have receded to prevent reoccurrence.

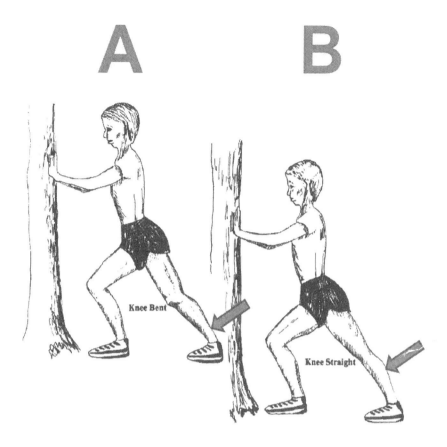

- **Figure A. Knee Bent**- the leg being stretched is the back one. The person is standing straight and bends both knees and at the same time she also bends her arms at the elbows towards the tree. The stretch should be felt at the bottom of the back of the lower leg (see arrow fig. A.)

- **Figure B. Knee Straight**- The leg being stretched is the back one. The person is leaning into the tree and just bends the front knee. The stretch should be felt in the middle to top of the calf muscle in the back leg (see arrow fig. B.)

- There is a stretch called the Plantar Fascial Stretch that we always recommend to be done for this condition.

- Sit on the floor or a bed and stretch your leg out with the knee straight in front of you.

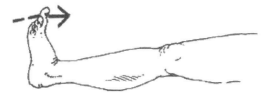

- Loop a towel or Theraband (elastic exercise band) around the bottom front of your foot and toes. Pull back with your arms as you stretch the foot and the toes back towards your face.

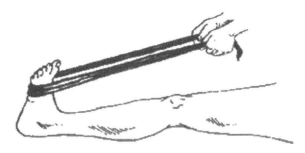

- Hold this for 30 seconds and repeat two to three times, two to three times a day.

14. **Plantar Fascial Braces** are used specifically to help stretch out the calf muscles. We usually recommend them for people who have chronic Plantar Fasciitis but in general they are very useful in getting the calf muscles stretched out. You cannot walk in them. You can sleep with them on. However, if you find that they interfere with your ability to sleep, you can put them on and use them for as long as you want during the day as long as you are able to stay off your feet. Follow the instructions that come with the braces on how to properly use them.

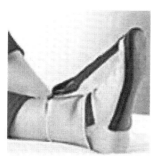

Foot Smart Brand-one example of many

When to Call the Doctor

If the pain and inflammation persists, does not respond at all, or gets worse after doing all the above, then you should seek professional care.

Practical Pointers for Prevention

- Stretching the calf and the foot should be done regularly.

- Wear good supportive shoes whenever you are going to be on your feet for long periods of time, and/or do a lot of walking.

- Wear the appropriate supportive sport specific shoes if you participate in sports/fitness activities regularly.

- Since this condition is often related to inefficient foot and leg functioning, make sure that you wear some arch supports, foot support insoles, or custom made orthotics that can help this condition.

- If you are overweight, then consider going on a weight loss and/or weight management program.

Pain in Bottom of Heel

Calcaneal Spur Syndrome, bursitis, nerve problems, stone bruises and stress fractures

What is it?

The following are several other conditions that can cause pain in the bottom of the heel which are more than skin deep. They have similar symptoms to and are often confused with plantar fasciitis (plantar fasciosis) though the differences between them are usually subtle.

The bad news is it could be difficult for you to figure out which one you have on your own.

The good news is that initially the treatment for all of these conditions is essentially the same (see pages 81-91).

Plantar Calcaneal Spur-is a shelf of bone, usually extending the entire width of the heel bone (Calcaneus) caused by excessive tension or pulling by the plantar fascia where it originates (attaches to) on the bottom of the heel bone.

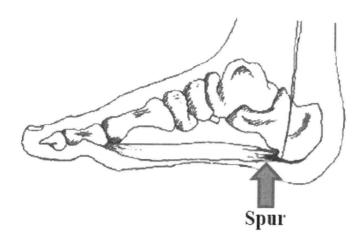

Spur

With plantar fasciitis there is pain, stiffness, and difficulty walking when one first gets out of bed in the AM or after sitting for long periods of time and standing up. With calcaneal spur syndrome, there is usually no pain on arising but as the day goes on it starts to build up.

Bursitis in the bottom of the heel is the formation of a protective sack of fluid, called a bursa, which can become painful when irritated and inflamed. The pain pattern is similar to the calcaneal spur syndrome but if the foot was x-rayed no bone spur would be found.

Nerve entrapment or compression (Baxter's Neuritis) is an entrapment or compression of a small nerve beneath the heel bone. The pain pattern is usually very similar to plantar fasciitis though, with Baxter's Neuritis there is usually no pain when getting out of bed in the morning. The pain starts with weight bearing activities and increases as the day goes on. There could also be burning, tingling, and numbness present which would not be the case with plantar fasciitis.

Tarsal Tunnel Syndrome-the tarsal tunnel is a narrow tunnel that is located behind the medial malleolus (the bump on the inside of the ankle bone). It houses a nerve, artery, veins, and several tendons. The nerve called the Posterior Tibial Nerve sometimes gets pinched (compressed) which can lead to heel pain. There may also be some sharp shooting type of pain and tingling in the heel that could also radiate into the arch and even extend up the lower leg.

Stone Bruise is defined as a contusion or injury to the soft tissue on the bottom of the heel. It is a painful injury caused by direct impact of a hard object or surface against the bottom of the heel of the foot. By its traumatic onset, it can usually be differentiated from these other problems. There is pain on weight bearing which can get progressively worse as the day goes on.

Calcaneal Stress Fractures-stress fractures are associated with tiny cracks that occur in bone due to repetitive stress over a period of time. This is usually related to an overuse type of injury associated with fitness activities such as: running, or walking, as well as overstressing the heel bone when doing an activity like dancing. You can often tell when someone has this type of injury, by cupping both the inside and outside of the heel in your hand and it will cause pain. The other heel problems mentioned will not have this same painful response. If you suspect this is what you have you should seek professional care.

Treatment

"Things you may need for treatment", "Preparation for treatment" and "Treatment" previously discussed in this chapter applies here (see pages 79-80).

Some "condition specific" recommendations are listed below.

For calcaneal spur syndrome and heel bursitis:

- You can pad the bottom of the heel to take stress off the painful area (spot).

- Cut a piece of adhesive backed ¼" felt or if you just have 1/8" adhesive backed felt, stick two pieces of it together and match it up to the size of the bottom your heel.

- Then locate the area on the bottom of the heel where the pain is and cut a hole in the heel pad so that the pressure can be removed from that spot.
- Some people prefer to make a donut shaped pad or "U" shaped pad instead.

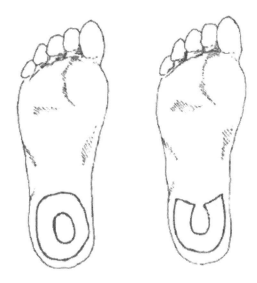

- Once you have the pad cut out and ready, use a tape adherent spray all around the bottom, back, and sides of the heel, going up about three inches or so from the bottom of the heel.
- Place the pad on the bottom of the foot.
- Then apply four 6" strips of 1&1/2" -2" adhesive tape to the pad as follows:
- Center one strip on the bottom of the heel pad and pull upward evenly on both sides, attaching them to the sides of the heel.

- Repeat with the second strip slightly behind the first, so that the bottom of the heel pad is covered.

- Center the third strip on the back of the heel (starting about one inch up from the bottom of the heel), pull around the heel and attach on the sides.

- Place the fourth strip so that it overlaps the third.

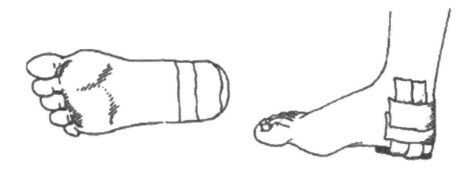

- This type of padding can be incorporated in the "low dye" taping technique as previously mentioned.

- As an alternative you can take an arch support or foot support insole and attach the heel pad to the bottom of it to take the pressure off the area as well. The pad may be more comfortable if it is shaved (skived down) using a scissor at an angle on the front of the pad.

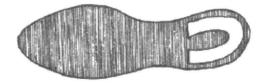

- Some people find relief also by using rubber or gel heel cups either with or without an arch support or foot support insole. If you want to do this as well, wear the heel cup over the arch support in your shoe.

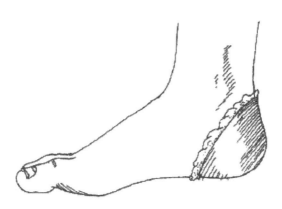

Remember, in both of these situations, whenever you add a heel raise or heel cup to an inlay, you should do so for both feet, unless you are compensating for a leg length discrepancy.

For a stone bruise, you can also use a heel pad as described above but you do not need to cut a hole in it and in addition, you can also use the heel cups as described above.

If you think you are dealing with a nerve problem and have tried all the treatment recommendations up to this point, then use a heating pad around the heel and ankle on medium heat two to three times daily for twenty minutes each time.

Make sure you put the heating pad around your ankle as well as your foot.

You can also take your arch support and add a "varus" wedge made of 1/8 inch adhesive foam or felt, to it.

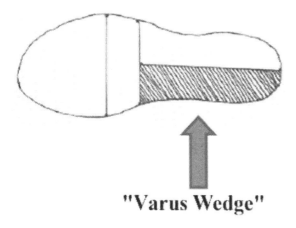

"Varus Wedge"

For a stress fracture of the heel, if you have tried all the treatment recommendations for 3-5 days with no results or it has gotten worse and the heel seems to hurt whenever you are on it, then do the squeeze test if you have not done it already. If you cup both the inside and outside of the heel in the palm of your hand and squeeze them together while off your foot and this causes you pain in that area, then you may have a stress fracture and should seek professional care.

When to call the Doctor

If the pain and inflammation persists or the area gets red, hot and/or swollen, does not respond at all, or gets worse after doing all the above, then you should seek professional care.

Practical Pointers for Prevention

- Stretching the calf and the foot should be done regularly.

- Wear good supportive shoes whenever you are going to be on your feet for long periods of time, and/or do a lot of walking.

- Don't use everyday shoes of more than 1 1/2" in heel height; they can cause havoc with your feet. If you have a heel problem and are stretching the back of your legs in order to alleviate it, the use of built-up heels in your everyday shoes will work against everything you are trying to accomplish with your stretching.

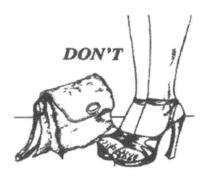

- Wear the appropriate supportive sport specific shoes if you participate in sports/fitness activities regularly. Since this condition is often related to inefficient foot and leg functioning, make sure that you wear some arch supports, foot support insoles, or custom made orthotics that can help this condition.

- If you are overweight, then consider going on a weight loss and/or weight management program.

11. DIABETES

Diabetes is the sixth leading cause of death in the United States, and approximately 20 million Americans have diabetes with an estimated 20 percent of the senior population age 60 and older being affected. Millions of people have diabetes and do not know it. Left undiagnosed, diabetes can lead to severe complications such as heart disease, stroke, blindness, kidney failure, leg and foot amputations, and death related to pneumonia and flu. Once you are diagnosed with diabetes, you already have many of these complications in place but just don't know it yet.

There are two types of diabetes.

Type 1 diabetes, predominantly occurs before the age of 20. You have to be on insulin for the rest of your life. The cause of type 1 is not entirely known. About 10 percent of all diabetics in the U.S. have type 1.

Persons with type 2 or adult-onset diabetes are commonly overweight and have high blood pressure and abnormal cholesterol levels at the time of diagnosis.

The incidence and prevalence of type 2 diabetes is skyrocketing around the world because if you have the genetic susceptibility for type 2, there are a couple of things that really bring it out: sedentary life style and obesity and because our society is getting heavier and less active, that's the main reason why we're seeing such a huge increase.

Scientific evidence now shows that early detection and treatment of diabetes with diet, physical activity, and new medicines can prevent or delay much of the illness and complications associated with diabetes.

Thousands of *people a day* in the United States are diagnosed with diabetes.

What is it?

Diabetes is a disease in which the body cannot properly utilize sugar intake. The sugar level builds up in the blood system and causes many negative changes. Diabetics are often more susceptible to infection, have problems in healing and circulatory disorders, especially in the feet.

Diabetics also have loss of sensitivity in the feet and thus ulcers, infections and injury may be present without their knowledge. For instance, in the case of many diabetics, ulcers develop on their feet that will ultimately lead to devastating complications and amputations. High blood sugar damages the nerve fibers in the feet causing **Diabetic Peripheral Neuropathy (DPN)**, the inability to feel to protect from injury, often resulting in both numbness and pain. This in itself is an enigma because these people have numb feet and yet they experience severe pain in them.

Here's how it works: If a non-diabetic has a pebble in his shoe, he will immediately feel it, take off his shoe and remove the pebble. If a diabetic with "DPN" has a pebble in his shoe he will continue to walk with it often not recognizing there is a problem until he or a family member notices blood and/or pus on the bathroom floor. Here is the timeline. It starts with a blister that becomes an ulcer and that gets infected. By the time the problem is noticed the person is on a downward slide from ulcer to infection and this often leads to amputations.

There are steps that can be taken and products that can be utilized to help a diabetic to predict, and thus prevent, even the first ulceration.

Preventing amputation in type 2 diabetes

Controlling ones blood sugar and **_checking your feet daily_** are *vital* to preventing the possibility of an amputation. However, if you've been told that you'll need an amputation then control of blood sugars may be impossible at that point.

Infections often play havoc with blood sugar control. At that point the ***doctor you choose to see may be the deciding factor.*** This often will be your primary care doctor if you have one.

If you don't have one going to an emergency room may be your only option. In addition to an emergency room doctor, other doctors who will be part of a team should be consulted.

A very important part of this team and often your best advocate is your podiatrist.

A podiatrist very often runs or is an integral part of the wound care center at your hospital.

He will know where you need to go. Also, if your circulation is impaired he will bring in a vascular surgeon who can bypass the blockage and increase the blood supply to the foot.

It is very important to understand this section. The wound care team consists of your podiatrist, infectious disease specialist, vascular surgeon and then surgeon, usually in that order. The surgeon is the last person you want to see when you have a foot or leg wound. The rest of the team includes your primary care doctor (internist) and other doctors dealing with any other complications you may have such as heart, eye, kidney disease and depression. 29% of diabetics suffer from depression and most don't know it. This often prevents them from properly caring for their issues.

It is certainly your best defense to try and prevent the doctor ever raising the possibility of amputation. Your best chance for that is tight control of your blood sugar.

Preventing wounds is your next best defense. Protecting your feet and if your feet develop wounds getting them promptly treated is the next best defense.

If you have a persistent wound that will not heal, don't accept that it is nothing to worry about. Seek another opinion!

It is extremely important for people who have diabetes to give special care to their feet.

The idea is to avoid rather than invite trouble that can lead to more serious problems; including gangrene, loss of toe(s), loss of limb and in many cases loss of life.

The average diabetic that has an amputation will live for two to five years because of the complications. There is hope however that one can beat these odds and live much longer if they become an active partner with their health care team and are willing to make some changes in their daily habits.

It is common knowledge that eating healthy foods and exercising are key factors in ensuring good health and can be effective in countering obesity that leads to type 2 diabetes.

Along with this, there are a variety of steps to take that may minimize its impact, particularly in decreasing the possibility of multiple hospitalizations, surgeries, and ultimately amputations.

The following are important recommendations for the foot care of diabetics.

ALL ARE NECESSARY!

Our goal for you in this section is education and prevention.

General Foot Hygiene for Diabetics

- Inspect your feet carefully, every day. Check the tops, bottoms (to see the bottom you will either need someone to look for you or you can get a mirror especially designed for this task), in-between your toes, and look over your toenails as well. Make sure you have no infection, redness, heat, swelling, pain, openings or ulcers, cuts, bruises, blisters, rashes, cracks, or newly opened areas producing pus and/or bleeding. Also note lumps, new corns or calluses. If you note any of these signs or anything unusual, consult your podiatrist or other healthcare professional immediately. If they are not readily available go to the emergency room at your local hospital.

- *Let the emergency room physician or your podiatrist care for you there and get the situation stabilized.*

- Wash your feet daily with warm water and soap. Be especially careful to clean between your toes. Try to use soaps that have glycerin in them as they are good for moisturizing the skin.

- **Be sure to check the temperature of the water by placing an elbow in it to make sure it is not too hot.**

- *Diabetics often cannot feel their feet and if the water is too hot are susceptible to scalding and burns.*

- Do not use any rubbing action what-so-ever on your feet and do not use very hot or very cold water.

- Dry them carefully, especially in between the toes. Do not rub with a coarse towel.

- Use a moisturizing cream on your feet both in the morning and at bedtime. For example, you can use a vegetable shortening or fifty-percent mixture of liquid Crisco oil and Vaseline, vitamin A cream, cocoa better, a good body cream or similar emollients.

- *If you are a DIABETIC you SHOULD NOT TREAT your own feet!*

- **If you have corns, callouses, nail problems, etc. the home care remedies suggested throughout this book are not for you.**

- Periodic, preventative visits to your podiatrist are strongly advised. The timing of these visits depends on the severity of your diabetes and what your podiatrist and or primary care physician recommends.

- We strongly advise Semmes-Weinstein *monofilament screening test* for Diabetic peripheral neuropathy on every diabetic whether they have yet developed diabetic peripheral neuropathy or not. A screening will give your doctors a baseline going forward so they can know whether the DPN is getting worse or not. Loss of feeling in the feet is often the start of the downward slide to ulcers, infections and amputation. Testing protective sensation on a regular basis is the key.

- The Semmes-Weinstein test uses a heavy nylon thread to touch specific areas of the bottom of each foot (circles). These monofilaments are readily available at your local pharmacy or online. You or someone in your household can easily learn to do this test and should a loss of sensation occur, contact your doctor immediately.

- A schematic of the test is shown here.

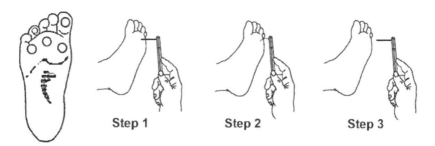

- It is important for all diabetics to have a conversation with their podiatrist or other healthcare provider about the Semmes-Weinstein test as well as other important screening tests for people who have diabetes including circulation, kidneys, eye exams and depression. If you don't already have a podiatrist as part of your healthcare team, get one.

- *If you have diabetes we do not even recommend you cut your own toenails.* However, if you insist and your hand is steady and your eyesight is still good (diabetes affects eyesight) and more importantly your blood sugar is under control (through a Hemoglobin A1c blood test) you can give it a try. Let us make ourselves perfectly clear, we still do not recommend it.

- Make sure that any instruments you use are clean. Wash them off with soap and water and rinse them off with alcohol or any recognized antiseptic solution. Make sure the materials and suggested medications are clean and up-to-date. A sterile gauze pad that has been sitting in a medicine cabinet for 5 years may no longer be sterile.

- Put two tablespoons of mild household detergent into 1 ½ gallons of *warm* water. Make sure you test the water temperature with your elbow before putting your feet into it. If you have diabetic peripheral neuropathy, and the water is too hot, you may burn yourself and not even know it.

- Dip your feet into the water and soak for ten minutes. Dry your feet thoroughly and gently with a soft towel especially between the toes. Apply an antiseptic solution or spray to the toenails.

- Trim and cut the toenails straight across. Always leave them a little longer than you think they should be cut.

- If you are in pain because of this, see a podiatrist immediately.

- After you have finished cutting your nails, rinse the toes off with warm soapy water. Dry your feet thoroughly and gently, especially between the toes. Apply an antiseptic liquid or spray.

- <u>*DO NOT ATTEMPT TO CUT INTO THE CORNERS OR DIG UNDER THE NAIL OR CUTICLE, NO MATTER WHAT!*</u>

- *Caution:* **We do not recommend you do this yourself. We know you are doing it, but we don't condone it. We prefer you have some professional guidance here. A simple slip could cost you a leg.**

- Most self-treatment for corns, callouses, hammertoes, warts, etc. is not recommended for diabetics. See a podiatrist!

- Similarly, any cuts, cracks, sores, abrasions and any other injuries should be treated only by a podiatrist or a doctor that knows something about treating diabetics.

- If you do sustain an injury, time is of the essence. See a doctor as soon as possible.

When attending to an injury situation (first aid) for a diabetic where the skin is torn, do the following:

- Wash the area carefully with soap and water.

- Make sure to remove all foreign material.

- Apply an antiseptic.

- Cover the wound with non-stick Adaptic (a non-adhering dressing material that won't stick to a wound) and then with a sterile gauze pad suited to the size of the problem (2X2, 3X3 etc.) and non-allergic paper tape.

- Call your podiatrist or primary care doctor.

- Never use over-the-counter medications such as medicated corn remedies unless prescribed by your podiatrist. These can cause serious problems even for people with healthy feet.

- If you have a problem with excessive foot perspiration, you may first try using a mild talcum powder on your feet and in your socks. However, if the problem still occurs, seek professional care.

- If for any reason you see the need to use tape on your feet without your doctors knowledge, do not use so-called regular adhesive-backed tape. Use the non-allergic tapes that peel away from the skin easily and are less abrasive to your skin.

Shoe--Do's and Don'ts for Diabetics

- Be careful in choosing shoe wear.

- Dress shoes should have soft leather uppers.

- Athletic shoes should have soft nylon uppers.

- Both types of shoes are less likely to irritate your feet, probably will conform easily to any lumps or bumps and will allow your feet to breathe properly.

- Do not choose shoes made of artificial upper material. They are not porous and are usually too stiff for proper comfort.

- Shoes must fit properly. They should not feel tight.

- Change shoes daily to allow them to dry out.

- Feet normally swell in the course of the day. Thus, it's best to shop for new shoes when feet are at their largest size, in the evenings.

- Be careful when buying high boots.

- Women's boots styles are especially likely to constrict the lower leg circulation of even people with healthy circulation. Diabetics should avoid these boots.

- *Diabetics should never, ever go barefoot. Use sandals, slippers, shower shoes or regular shoes.*

Hosiery--Do's and Don'ts for Diabetics

- Wear properly fitted socks.

- Don't wear tube socks that are supposedly made to fit several foot sizes.

- Don't wear socks with tight-elastic top bands.

- Don't wear non-prescribed support hose because they may be too constrictive.

- The best socks are wool, cotton or nylon blended socks.

- Socks should be clean and changed daily.

- Don't wear hosiery that needs to be mended. The mending will often lead to the formation of seams that can be irritating. This is especially dangerous for diabetics.

- Don't wear anything tight around the legs or ankles that might interfere with the circulation to your feet.

- Don't wear restrictive circular-shaped socks or hose.

General Health Considerations for Diabetics...

- Keep blood sugar, blood pressure, and cholesterol levels under control.

- Eat healthy and avoid sugar, fried foods, alcohol, tobacco and bad carbohydrates. Learn to read labels. For example many of the foods we enjoy have *high fructose corn syrup* in them. This stuff is poison for staying healthy and especially for diabetics. Avoid it!

- Learn how to calculate your body mass index and keep it below 25.

- Keep your waist size below 40.

- Exercise regularly for 30 minutes, 5-7 days a week.

- Especially on days that end in "y".

- *The best amputation prevention is prevention.*

- *Make sure you keep appointments with your team of doctors- primary care, podiatrist, vascular, eye, kidney, heart, mental health, dentist, etc.*

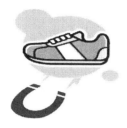
Several years ago we came across an alternative and complementary, non-medical solution that your doctor may not be familiar with and perhaps you need to know about!

- A ground breaking research study was published that could provide a ray of hope for diabetics suffering from diabetic peripheral neuropathy (DPN). The study, "Static Magnetic Field Therapy for Symptomatic Diabetic Neuropathy: A Randomized, Double-Blind, Placebo-Controlled Trial", by Michael I. Weintraub, MD, FACP, FAAN, et al, published in the May, 2003, issue of the Archives of Physical Medicine and Rehabilitation, broke new ground.

- The study concluded the following... "Although many questions remain about a precise mechanism of action, the present study provides convincing data confirming that the constant wearing of static, permanent, magnetic insoles produces statistically significant reduction of neuropathic pain. Considering their safety and minimal cost (<$100) our data suggest that the insoles may be used as adjunctive or monotherapy. Future studies are needed to identify the optimal time to achieve maximum antinociceptive effect and to confirm and extend these results. Additional search for biologic markers (i.e., epidermal nerve fiber biopsy, microneurography) will be necessary in future protocols to determine if permanent structural changes can be produced."

- Reduction of Diabetic Neuropathy, by any means, will considerably curtail the need for amputations in the diabetic population thus potentially saving thousands of limbs and subsequently thousands of lives.

Disclaimer: "This material has been produced by Dr. Mark D. Sussman and Dr. Myles J. Schneider, Independent Nikken Consultants, and is not official material prepared or provided by Nikken, Inc."

12. FOOT & ANKLE INJURY

What to Do If You Get Hurt

R. I. C. E.

This stands for: rest, ice, compression, and elevation. It is often used after acute injury or for painful conditions for the first 48-72 hours to reduce pain, swelling, and inflammation.

Rest

In the treatment of painful conditions, rest can be achieved in several different ways:

- It can mean pursuing all normal daily activities except those that put severe stress on the area (such as the stress of athletic training).
- It can mean substituting one activity for another (as in riding a bicycle or swimming instead of running).
- It can mean putting partial weight on the painful part by using a cane to get around with.
- It can also mean using a walking cast, or putting no weight on the painful part (crutch walking).
- In an extreme case, it can also mean complete bed rest.

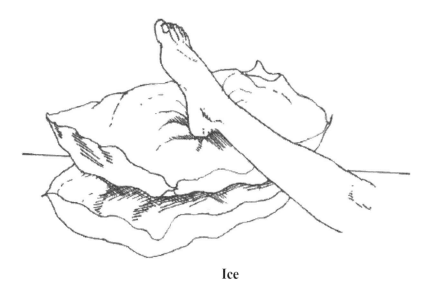

Ice

Cold (ice) therapy is used for acute injuries because it decreases swelling, tissue damage, and inflammation.
- **It should not be used where there is decreased sensation or numbness.**
- **It should not be used in people who have poor circulation, circulatory disease or circulatory conditions like Reynaud's Phenomenon or Reynaud's disease which is more serious.**
- **Though not very common, it should not be used if someone has a known allergy to ice which is manifested by hives (red, bumpy, blotches or welts that are usually itchy and the foot can become swollen as well).**

How to make it up...

- Ice bags are most commonly used.
- Or use a cold pack.
- Or use a towel covering a plastic bag filled with crushed ice.
- Or use a frozen bag of vegetables (this works well).
- Or fill a paper cup with water and freeze it into an easy-to-use ice applicator.
- Or if you have a home whirlpool or Jacuzzi use cold water in them.

Some examples are shown here:

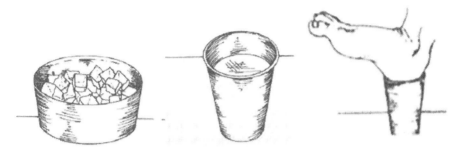

How to use ...

- Apply to the affected area for 10- 20 minutes at least three times a day when possible for the first 48 -72 hours.
- The 10-20 minutes range here is used because thinner people may not be able to tolerate the cold as well as a heavier person. There are four stages that cold therapy goes through. They are: discomfort, stinging, burning, and finally numbness. Dependent on the size of the person and the part of the body being iced, the stages can be reached within 5 – 15 minutes.
- Once you think you have gone through the four stages, then try and keep the ice on for another 5 minutes.
- **If you have any doubts and/or are concerned that it is too uncomfortable and/or too cold, then stop and rest the area for at least 20 minutes and try it again. It is better to be safe than sorry.**
- Ice packs should be used with caution. They should be wrapped in a towel before being placed on and/or around the affected area.
- If you purchase some type of ice pack, bag, or other cold producing modality, follow the instructions carefully. Ice used improperly or too long can irritate and damage the skin and the tissue below.
- Some people are allergic to ice. If this is the case, then the area involved will break out in hives as described above. If you are one of these people or this happens to you for the first time, try to go somewhere where it is warm and place the foot in warm water and seek professional care. Obviously, it would behoove you not to use ice or cold therapy in the future unless told differently by your doctor.

Compression

- The purpose of compression is to control/limit swelling, give support to the injured part, decrease pain and stimulate/speed up healing and recovery.
- Whenever using this form of treatment on the foot, you should wrap the entire foot from the toes to above the calf muscle using a 2" or 3" Ace bandage. If you do it just to cover a smaller injured area, you will see swelling seeping through the end of the wrap and by covering the entire foot and lower leg you will be better able to give support to all the musculoskeletal tissues in the area (muscles, joints, ligaments, tendons).
- The wrap should be comfortable.
- It should be kept in place ideally for the first 10-12 hours if possible.
- Ice can be placed over the compression wrap as needed.

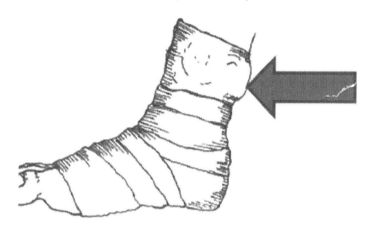

- Place 2-4 large gauze pads against the skin to protect it from frostbite. A plastic baggie filled with ice is put against these pads and wrapped with an ACE bandage.
- **If the foot becomes numb, tingles, or the toes start to get blanched (pale) looking, blue, and/or cold, then the bandage may be wrapped too tightly. Unwrap it for a several hours and wiggle your toes and move your foot gently (so as not to cause you too much pain from the injury) for the first few minutes, then rewrap the foot a little looser this time.**

Elevation

- This will help reduce swelling and pain. If too much fluid rushes to and accumulates in an injured area it can cause pressure to the nerves and other tissues in the area, leading to increased pain and potentially can delay healing.

- The foot and lower leg should be elevated on two pillows so that it is elevated above the level of the heart. This should be done as much as possible over the first 48 hours or can be discontinued sooner if you wish, once the throbbing stops when lowering your leg.

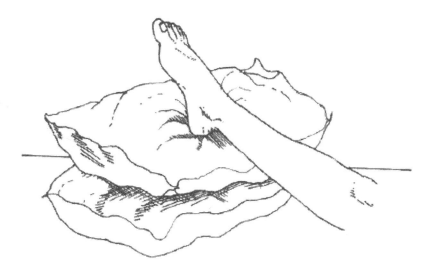

Heat

- Increasing the temperature to a part of the body that has been injured can help reduce muscle tension, decrease stiffness, and promote healing by increasing the circulation.

- **Unless told differently by a healthcare professional, heat is not usually indicated for new injuries for at least the first 48 hours.**
- **Heat should not be used over an area that is already red unless told to by a healthcare professional.**

- **You should not use heat on an area of your body that has lost some of its sensation or is numb. Applying heat to the injured area is usually recommended *after* the first 48 hours.**

There are several ways that you can apply heat to the affected area.

- Moist heating pads are probably the best way to do this. They work better than regular dry heating pads. Moist heat has better penetration then dry heat. It also will not dehydrate the area you are heating and this is better for stimulating the circulation. We would recommend using the low to medium intensity settings on the heat control button.
- You can also use hot water bottles as well as hot packs.
- If you are going to use dry heat packs, then cover with a warm, moist, towel.
- You can also fill up a bath tub with warm to hot water.
- Whichever way you use for heat, follow the directions on the product you have purchased.
- If you have a home whirlpool bath or Jacuzzi, use warm water (ninety to one hundred degrees Fahrenheit).
- The heat should be applied twenty minutes on and then off for at least twenty minutes, if you intend to apply it repeatedly. Otherwise, we recommend using heat for twenty minutes at least two to three times a day.
- Depending on the type of problem you have, massaging the affected part is often recommended just after heating it.
- *Do not fall asleep when using heating pads and remember to make sure you do not apply heat for more than twenty minutes at a time. Do not use an electric heating pad while soaking in a bathtub or when soaking your feet in a basin of water.*

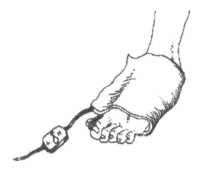

- There are a variety of over-the-counter products that can produce heat to an area like Ben Gay and Icy Hot (these are two of several available.

  We don't recommend one over the other.

  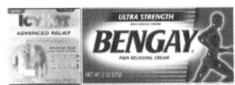

  Make sure you use as directed.

- If you are not sure about how to use these types of products or have any questions, ask your pharmacist and/or your doctor for guidance.
- The following information should be included with your instructions but is very important so we will mention them here:
  Do not apply more then 3-4 times per day.
  Do not apply on open cuts or wounds.
  Do not apply heat inducing topical medication and then cover with a tight wrap or bandage because it can generate too much heat, burn and/or irritate the skin. You can cover the foot with a loose cloth or one of your socks.
  Do not apply and then immediately cover it with a heating pad.
  Wash your hands immediately and thoroughly after application to the injured area.

- **Do not place heating pads over an area after applying such a product. This could cause burn damage to the skin.**

Ice and Heat

Ice is recommended for at least the first 48 hours and then often heat afterwards (there is some controversy about this among certain ancillary health practitioners but this is what we recommend) however some people find that one modality works best for them or makes them feel better than another. If you find that using heat after the first 48 hours does not seem to help but continued use of cold does, then do what works best for you.

Contrast Baths (Hot and Cold Therapy)

Contrast baths involve submerging a part of the body in warm to hot water for a few minutes and then immediately placing the same part in cold water for a few minutes. This process is repeated several times. This type of therapy has been reported to increase the circulation to an area and stimulate the lymphatic system which can expedite healing.

- Place warm to slightly hot (not scalding) water in a basin or tub that you can soak your foot in. In an adjacent basin or tub place some cold water with some ice cubes in it.
- Submerge the injured foot in the warm to hot water first for 2 minutes and then immediately take it out and place it in the cold water for 2 minutes. While the foot is in either tub you can move it around (up and down in and out) to pain tolerance.
- This procedure is repeated 3 times in succession and should be done at least once a day. If you choose to do it more than once daily, then doing this contrast bath therapy up to three times a day (morning, afternoon, and evening or night time) should be sufficient.
- This can be repeated daily until the pain is gone and the injury is healed.
- Some people like to also use it after fitness/athletic activities even after recovering from an injury and that is certainly okay to do.
- Others who are not into fitness/athletic activities and no longer have pain or any other symptoms, related to their injury, feel this is beneficial to them. Therefore, at the end of a busy day, especially when they have been on their feet an extended period of time, they enjoy using this contrast bath therapy.

Over-the- Counter Medications

There are some over-the-counter, non-steroidal, anti-inflammatory medications that help reduce pain, swelling, and inflammation. Some of these are: Advil, Aleve, Motrin, and Naproxen.

- Tylenol can be used to reduce the pain but it does not have the same anti-inflammatory properties as the above do.
- Always take these as directed.
- Never take more than the recommended dosages.
- Do not take more than one type of these at a time.
- Do not take aspirin if you are already taking one of these.
- Do not drink alcohol with them.
- Make sure you read all the information especially about: side effects, special warnings, food and drug interactions, and information concerning pregnancy and/or breast feeding.
- These types of medications taken for a prolonged period can be very harmful to you. Therefore, do not use them more then you need to. In addition, if you have no results within ten days stop taking them and then consider some other treatment or seek professional care.
- If after ten days you only notice relief of your pain when using the medication and you do not really notice any progress other than that, then you should seek professional care as well.

When to call the doctor

1. If swelling persists, recurs with walking or is present after a few days, rest and seek professional care.

2. Also, seek care when any injury accompanied by severe pain does not resolve itself within a few days.

3. Any area where there is pus, heat, persistent swelling and/or redness, chills and fever (the signs of infection) should also be checked by a doctor.

4. If you think a joint is involved with your injury, see a doctor.

Don't be a hero. If for any reason you feel that you would like to have something checked out by a doctor, you should definitely have it done.

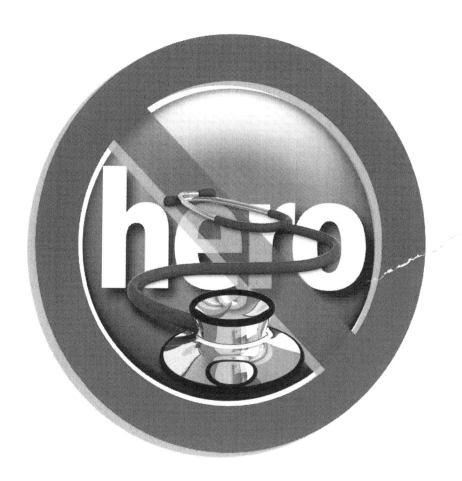

Acknowledgements

Our thanks to Steve Wright of QuickPro Graphics whose tireless design work and all around assistance proved over and over again he was the right man for the job.

Special thanks to Brian Sussman of Sussman Multimedia for his technical support when it was desperately needed.

About the Authors

Doctors Schneider & Sussman featured in

"People Magazine"

October 26, 1981

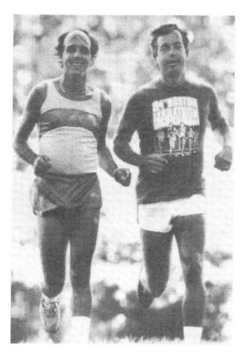

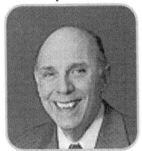

Dr. Myles J. Schneider grew up in the Bronx, New York and graduated from New York University with a B.A. degree. He received his degree in Podiatric Medicine (DPM) from the Kent State University College of Podiatric Medicine-formerly the Ohio College of Podiatric Medicine and did his specialty training in Foot and Ankle Surgery at the Kern Hospital for Special Surgery in Detroit, Michigan. He is a Diplomate of the American Board of Podiatric Medicine and a Fellow of the American College of Foot and Ankle Orthopedics and Medicine. He has been in private practice for over 40 years, currently at the Annandale Foot and Ankle Center in Annandale, Virginia. His special interests include podiatric sports medicine and biomechanics. He co-authored 3 books with Dr. Mark Sussman, including the international best seller, *How to Doctor Your Feet Without the Doctor*, Charles Scribner and Sons, New York, NY, 1981. His most recent book is, *To Be or Not to Be Healthy-For Most of Us this is a Choice.* Dr. Schneider's future plans are to devote as much time as he can, offering information on the importance of everyone becoming proactive and responsible for their own health.

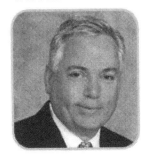

Dr. Mark D. Sussman is a native Washingtonian (DC). He received his degree in Podiatric Medicine (DPM) from the Kent State College of Podiatric Medicine-formally the Ohio College of Podiatric Medicine and did his specialty training in Foot and Ankle Surgery at the Kern Hospital for Special Surgery in Detroit, Michigan. He is a Diplomate of The American Board of Podiatric Surgery and a Fellow of the American College of Foot and Ankle Surgeons. He is a Founding Member *Emeritus* of the American Society of Podiatric Surgeons. He co-authored 3 books with Dr. Myles Schneider, including the international best seller, *How to Doctor Your Feet Without the Doctor*, Charles Scribner and Sons, New York, NY, 1981. His latest book, *How Emily's Sick House Got Well and So Did Her Family,* is a fable introducing children to the world of wellness. Mark practiced in Wheaton, Maryland for 31 years, specializing in Foot Surgery. He retired from his practice in 2001.

Mark D. Sussman, DPM and Myles J. Schneider, DPM

Contacting the Authors

For more information on ordering additional copies of this book or any other books by the authors, including e-Books visit our website. There is a wealth of information, self-help tips and links to additional resources and much more.

In addition, if you or someone else has questions or concerns about foot problems, please visit our website and use our contact form and we will respond as quickly as possible.

www.MSFootDoctors.com

Made in the USA
San Bernardino, CA
27 July 2015